A Handbook of Essential Drugs and Regimens in Hematological Oncology

A Handbook of Essential Drugs and Regimens in Hematological Oncology

AARON POLLIACK M.D.
Professor of Medicine and Hematology
Head of Lymphoma-Leukemia Unit
Haematology Department
Hadassah University Hospital
Hebrew University-Hadassah Medical School
Jerusalem, Israel

harwood academic publishers
chur · reading · paris · philadelphia · tokyo · melbourne

Harwood Academic Publishers

Post Office Box 90
Reading, Berkshire RG1 8JL
United Kingdom

58, rue Lhomond
75005 Paris
France

5301 Tacony Street, Drawer 330
Philadelphia, Pennsylvania 19137
United States of America

3-14-9, Okubo
Shinjuku-ku, Tokyo 169
Japan

Private Bag 8
Camberwell, Victoria 3124
Australia

Library of Congress Cataloging-in-Publication Data

Polliack, Aaron, 1939-
A handbook of essential drugs and regimens in hematological oncology / by Aaron Polliack.
p. cm.
Includes bibliographical references and indexes.
ISBN 3-7186-5096-7 (hard). -- ISBN 3-7186-5097-5 (soft)
1. Leukemia--Chemotherapy--Handbooks, manuals, etc.
2. Lymphoma--Chemotherapy--Handbooks, manuals, etc.
3. Antineoplastic agents--Handbooks, manuals, etc.
I. Title. II. Title: Essential drugs and regimens in hematological oncology.
[DNLM: 1. Anti-Neoplastic Agents--therapeutic use--handbooks.
2. Leukemia--drug therapy--handbooks. 3. Lymphoma--drug therapy--handbooks. QV 39 P774h]
RC643.P62 1991
616.99'419061--dc20
DNLM/DLC
For Library of Congress 91-20860
CIP

 Printed in the United Kingdom by Bell and Bain Ltd.

CONTENTS

PREFACE

During more than twenty years of experience in hematological oncology, I have felt an increasing need for a practical 'pocket' handbook to assist the staff treating patients with these disorders. This handbook contains basic information relating to the administration of cytotoxic drugs, details of the chemotherapeutic agents frequently used, tabulation of their common side-effects, and details of the regimens most commonly used in the treatment of myelomas, leukemias and lymphomas. Staff treating patients with these disorders could then easily refer to the contents during their busy daily routine. Following discussions with many doctors involved in the treatment of these patients in general hospitals and specific cancer centers, I have become even more convinced that such a handbook would be most useful both for young and for more experienced physicians who often used to refer to a particular drug or protocol before using them in their daily practice. The nursing staff and pharmacists, who are just as involved in the treatment of patients with these disorders as the physicians, could also use it in their work.

Obviously, this is a dynamic rapidly changing field of medicine, and newly discovered chemotherapeutic agents and alternative regimens and protocols are being added all the time. Nevertheless, certain basic premises continue to form the backbone for therapy and older 'vintage' drugs with proven efficacy, utilized in what may now be considered more conventional and well-established regimens, continue to be used in the therapy of these disorders despite the fact that new agents and regimens have been introduced. These drugs and many of the regimens containing these agents are listed in this handbook as well as the established conventional agents and successful regimens which will always be considered for use in the treatment of hematological oncologic disorders. Current alternatives to these established drug combinations, utilizing new drugs and combination regimens, are also listed, as are some of the newer protocols used for cytoreduction prior to autologous bone-marrow transplantation; however, these may still have to stand the test of time in the treatment of hematological neoplasias.

The introductory section deals with the administration and general aspects of chemotherapeutic agents, including toxicity and side-effects. This is followed by a larger chapter, part 1, listing the anticancer drugs generally used in hemato-oncology, and which also provides brief notes on their mechanism of action, routine dosages and common side-effects. The Appendix to Part 1 includes tables with definitions of performance status and response criteria which are important in routine work. Finally, Part 2 lists many of the protocols used in the treatment of these disorders.

It is hoped that this handbook will be of assistance to all physicians, nurses and staff involved in the treatment of unfortunate patients with these neoplastic disorders in hospitals and day-care centers.

Acknowledgement

This handbook was prepared with the help of Timothy Root, Head of Pharmacy, The Royal Marsden Hospital, London, Fulham Road, UK. I am deeply grateful for his important contributions.

LIST OF DRUGS

Generic name (synonym) [Trade name]

Actinomycin D (Dactinomycin) [Cosmegen Lyorac]
Adrenal corticosteroids – prednisolone, prednisone, dexamethasone
Amsacrine (*m*-AMSA) [Amsidine]
L-Asparaginase [Elspar]
5-Azacytidine

Bleomycin [Blenoxane]
Busulfan [Myleran]

Carboplatin (Cis-dichloro cyclobutane, dicarboxylato platinum) [Paraplatin, CBDCA, JM-8]
Carmustine (BCNU) [BiCNU]
CCNU (lomustine)
Chlorambucil [Leukeran]
2-Chlorodeoxyadenosine
Cisplatin (cis-platinum, Cis – DDP, CDDP) [Neoplatin, Platinex, Platinol]
Cyclophosphamide [Endoxane, Cytoxan, Neosar]
Cytosine arabinoside (cytarabine) [Cytosar, Alexan]

Dacarbazine [DTIC]
Daunorubicin (daunomycin, rubidomycin) [Cerubidin]
Deoxycoformycin (DCF) [Pentostatin]
Doxorubicin [Adriamycin]

Epirubicin [Pharmorubicin]
Etoposide (VP-16) [Vepesid]

Fludarabine phosphate
5-Fluorouracil (5FU)

Hydroxyurea [Hydrea]

Idarubicin [Zavedos]
Ifosfamide [Mitoxana, Holoxan]
Interferon (IFN) [Intron – A, Roferon, Wellferon]

Interleukin-2 (IL-2)

Mechlorethamine (nitrogen mustard)
6-Mercaptopurine (6-MP) [Purinethol]
MESNA (Na-2-mercapto-ethane-sulfonate) [Vromitexan]
Methotrexate (MTX)
Methylhydrazine (procarbazine) [Matulan, Matulane]
Methyl GAG (mitoguazone)
Mithramycin [Mithracin]
Mitoxantrone [Novantrone]

Rubidazone

Streptozotocin [Zanosar]

Teniposide (VM-26) [Vumon]
6-Thioguanine (6-TG) [Lanvis]
Thiotepa

Vinblastine [Velbe]
Vincristine [Oncovin]
Vindesine [Eldesine]

ABBREVIATIONS

ADH, anti-diuretic hormone
ALL, acute lymphoblastic leukemia
AML, acute myeloid leukemia
ANLL, acute non-lymphoblastic leukemia
Ara-C, cytosine arabinoside

BMT, bone-marrow transplantation
BUN, blood urea nitrogen

CLL, chronic lymphocytic leukemia
CML, chronic myeloid leukemia
CR, complete remission

DN, deoxynucleotide

IC, intracavitory
ID, intradermal
IL-2, interleukin-2
IM, intramuscular
IT, intrathecal
i.u., international unit
IV, intravenous

LAK, lymphokine-activated killer

PO, per os
PR, partial remission

SC, subcutaneous
SGOT, serum glutamic oxaloacetic transaminase

TIL, tumor-infiltrating lymphocytes
TNF, tumor necrosis factor

WBC, white blood cell

PRACTICAL GUIDE TO THE USE OF CYTOTOXIC DRUGS

INTRODUCTION

Antineoplastic agents are almost only used in the treatment of histologically proven neoplasias. The majority of these drugs are cell poisons and their therapeutic efficiency is dangerously close to their toxicity. In addition to their effect on tumor cells, these agents will also affect many of the rapidly growing normal tissues which have a quick turnover in the body. These include hair follicles, gastrointestinal mucosa, cells of the reproductive system and hematopoietic tissue, resulting in side-effects commonly encountered clinically. Some agents will also concentrate selectively in certain tissues and their action will then be directed against these cells causing specific toxicity and serious injury in these particular organs. Furthermore, if these agents are used in an inappropriate manner severe life-threatening toxicity and even death may occur. However, when the physician is aware of these potential and expected side-effects, chemotherapy can be used effectively with an expected degree of minimal or moderate toxicity.

In principle, during therapy, patients must be forewarned of the expected toxicity and side-effects which may occur regularly with a particular drug which they are receiving. A simple example of this may be the sudden appearance of alopecia in a patient who was not warned of this complication beforehand. This event may prove upsetting to the individual concerned, unpleasant for both the patient and the doctor, eventually affecting the relationship that has developed between them. Sometimes physicians prescribe drugs without describing the expected side-effects to the patient or his family and this situation obviously must be avoided. Thus, explanations and discussions with patients receiving chemotherapy are essential, appropriate and correct. On the other hand, one could also argue that it may not be necessary to describe in full detail all the complex and rare side-effects of each drug to all patients and some of this information may best be imparted to family. In this respect medico-legal aspects have also become of prime importance in certain countries, particularly when patients have to give consent or signed agreement for the use of certain drugs. These factors may force the physician to impart unpleasant and frightening information to the patient prior to the therapy, and the manner and style to be employed in these discussions obviously depends on the individual physician concerned. Some doctors will no doubt succeed better than others in this respect.

The physician using chemotherapy must be guided by certain basic rules which must be strictly adhered to prior to beginning any therapy. Obviously antineoplastic agents should never be administered if the treating physician (1) is not aware of the potential side-effects or has never used the agent before without proper instruction, (2) has any question concerning the correct dose required to be given, (3) has no means of monitoring toxicity in an acceptable fashion, (4) does not have parameters to measure objective response or (5) lacks the results of basic blood tests required to determine drug dosage, or has results which may in fact constitute a contra-indication to the administration of the drug concerned.

It is important to remember that once these drugs have been administered there is, in most cases, no antedote to neutralize their actions or to prevent serious immediate or delayed side-effects. If the physician is in any way hesitant to treat for any of the above reasons, it is best not to administer the drug at all.

Prior to administration of any chemotherapy, full blood counts must be available so as to avoid giving the drug to a patient with unexpected low counts. Blood biochemistry results are also vital, in order to avoid administration of the agent in the presence of possible metabolic upsets such as incipient renal or liver failure, hypercalcemia, hyperuricemia and hyperglycemia, all of which may immediately compromise the health and the optimal response to chemotherapy. Many of these upsets may have to be corrected prior to administration of the drug.

TOXICITY AND EXTRAVASATION

GENERAL COMMENTS

In general, toxicity is dependent on the agent administered; however, in most cases, drugs are given until a recognized side-effect occurs, which may limit its further use during therapy. For example, alopecia, minor mucositis, nausea, vomiting and skin pigmentation are all side-effects which are expected to occur but are not generally drug-limiting.

On the other hand, thrombocytopenia, leukopenia, severe anemia, gastrointestinal bleeding, severe mucositis with oral ulcerations, pulmonary fibrosis and even severe diarrhea are all examples of drug-limiting toxicity. While clinical responses occur with some drugs without reaching toxicity, most hemato-oncologists will continue to use these agents optimally, until an acceptable degree of toxicity develops before stopping the drug, thereby ensuring that an adequate trial of the agent has been given, before therapy is altered. Certain agents given by the intravenous (IV) route are particularly irritating and may cause local reactions when inadvertent extravasation occurs into the subcutaneous tissues. Severe pain, erythema and ulcerations can occur after spillage, particularly with agents like vinblastine, vincristine and doxorubicin, therefore, great care should be taken to avoid extravasation. Obviously, aseptic techniques should be adhered to throughout. Experience has shown that certain techniques can be utilized to minimize extravasation of drugs and these include the following:

1. For direct infusion IV, a butterfly-type device should always be used which provides for easy change of syringes, simple insertion and greater safety. The device also has the advantage of being able to be used for multiple injections.

2. For continuous infusions, a small cannula may be used with greater safety. All these should be as small as possible and a 22/23 gauge is usually sufficient, causing minimal trauma.

3. Drugs are easily administered through a running IV infusion. When adding any drug to an IV solution or infusion set, a new sterile needle should always be used, preferably a 22/23 gauge type which will cause only minimal trauma. A small needle also

prevents administration too rapidly, provides for quick dilution of the drug and, in case of extravasation, ensures that only a small amount of drug will be injected outside the vein.

4. The vein to be used should be superficial, easily visible, as straight as possible and preferably unused. Previously bruised or inflamed areas and any limb with compromised circulation should be avoided. Limbs with obvious phlebitis, trauma, lymphedema, post-mastectomy or venous obstruction should obviously not be used. Veins on the dorsum of the hand are preferable for they are generally easily accessible and visible, and if any extravasation occurs, it will be rapidly noted in this area.

5. It is generally accepted that one person should *not try* to insert the infusion more than three times. Thereafter a second person with more experience should attempt insertion.

6. Prior to administration of the drug, the flow should be tested in the vein using normal saline and, of course, the vein should be well-flushed after infusion. If multiple drugs are to be given in the same set, the veins should be flushed between each administration. If the vein is fragile or small, the best procedure would be to attach the IV device to a normal saline infusion using an intermittent flushing technique; alternatively, if the vein is large enough, a fast-running infusion can be used, into which the drug can be given simultaneously.

7. When different drugs are prescribed, any drug which is a vesicant should be administered first, because the integrity of the vein will be optimal at that particular moment and extravasation is least likely.

8. Care should always be taken to ensure that all the drug enters the vein because many of the drugs with potential vesicant effect can cause extreme damage to the vein if leakage occurs. Because even small leaks are dangerous, one must always check for a ready backflow of blood at short intervals. If there is any doubt about leakage, it is preferable to stop the infusion immediately.

9. Drugs kept in the refrigerator will cause a cold sensation and this phenomenon should be distinguished from the burning sensation indicative of extravasation. If, after repeated injections or phlebitis, certain veins become sensitive, it is recommended that

they be flushed more frequently with saline, injected very slowly, using a smaller gauge needle (if possible a 25 gauge winged device) and preferably, inserted into a fast-running infusion.

10. Following injection, the arm should not be folded as this may result in relative venostasis, resulting in possible leakage of drug back through the injection site. It may also increase exposure of the vein to the drug locally, thereby enhancing local phlebitis and premature obliteration of the vein. Preferably, the patient should keep the arm straight for 2 min following injection of the drug with light pressure applied through an alcohol sponge.

MANAGEMENT OF EXTRAVASATION

Many drugs are vesicant and leakage can cause initial phlebitis, followed by severe ulceration and necrosis. If any doubt arises concerning venous patency or a potential leakage, stop the injection immediately and restart it in the other arm, or at least in a vein proximal to the previous puncture site.

Signs of extravasation include the following: a sharp burning sensation or stinging in the needle puncture area is felt by the patient; no return of blood is evident to the physician when the syringe is pulled back. Alternatively resistance may be felt on the syringe plunger during bolus administration, lack of free flow is seen if an infusion is in progress, swelling or leakage may be detected at the site of puncture.

In the presence of extravasation —*stop administration immediately, withdraw* the solution by *pulling back on the syringe* and remove the needle. *Cover the area with a cold ice-pack.* Inject hydrocortisone (100–200 mg) or dexamethasone (4 mg) around the entire area of extravasation subcutaneously (SC) or intradermally (ID) using a 25 gauge needle. Apply 1 % hydrocortisone cream and cover the site with an ice-pack for 24 h. Continue using the hydrocortisone ointment twice daily until the redness disappears.

Some suggest an injection of 5 ml of 1 % lignocaine (xylocaine 50 mg in the area). However, this decision must only be made by the treating physician. Once treated, the patient must watch for the development of subsequent blisters and ulcers and report to the treating physician for further follow-up.

SAFETY AND PROTECTIVE MEASURES

The Pharmacy is the best environment for reconstituting drugs, in a vertical laminar airflow safety cabinet which protects the drugs from microbial contamination. This constitutes the safest way of handling cytotoxic drugs as well as minimizing the potential hazards to pharmacy staff. If drugs are reconstituted in a ward or out-patient day hospital clinic facility, one should ideally wear glasses or goggles, gloves, a surgical mask and a plastic apron, while preparing the solution.

WARNINGS FOR ORAL AGENTS

Do not give prescriptions for a large amount of the oral drug to out-patients. Some of these drugs may get to be beyond their expiry date and the possibility of inadvertent or deliberate over-dosage is always present. If a patient is taking multiple agents, it is preferable to write out an explanatory schedule indicating the times that medication should be taken.

Certain oral alkylating agents may cause abdominal distress. In order to decrease these symptons, it is sometimes possible to divide the total dose into several portions or to recommend taking the entire dose at bedtime. Anti-emetic compounds are always used but these may not be completely effective.

SIDE-EFFECTS OF CYTOTOXIC DRUGS

GENERAL COMMENTS

Full details of side-effects for all specific drugs will be provided in the next chapter, however some very general comments are given below.

Gastrointestinal symptoms, particularly nausea and vomiting or diarrhea, are generally due to the effect of chemotherapy upon the central nervous system. Therefore, sedative anti-emetics are most useful to prevent these manifestations. Premedication should be given about 2–3 h before the IV administration of drugs and thereafter during 24 h. If severe diarrhea is expected, antispasmodic medications may be given. Patients should be advised not to drive or work until the effects of the anti-emetics have worn off. See further comments on anti-emetics on page 12.

MYELOSUPPRESSION

This occurs after most cytotoxic agents are given and the next batch of chemotherapy can be given in its full dose only after a full blood count has been performed. If the counts are not normal, drug dosage must be attenuated, according to the general scheme given below or alternatively, delayed until full recovery of the blood counts occurs. Since chemotherapy is most effective when given in full dosage, it is probably advisable to attempt to lengthen the interval between courses rather than to reduce the dosage after myelosuppression. In general, patients should remain at home when the counts are low, rather than in hospital, because in principle home-acquired sepsis may be less virulent and is easier to control and treat than that acquired in a hospital environment. Immunosuppressed patients with low white blood cell (WBC) counts should avoid contact with people who have known infections and it is also preferable to avoid crowded places. Repeated platelet tranfusions are given if there is bleeding or when the platelet count is less than 20×10^9/l. Antibiotic regimens are indicated when the fever rises over 38 °C and particularly in the presence of neutropenia or agranulocytosis while red blood cells are given if there is severe symptomatic anemia. Apart from the above-mentioned general side-effects, certain agents will have toxicity in specific tissues and these are dealt with in Part 1 where individual drugs are discussed e.g. cardiotoxicity, most frequently encountered with some anthracyclines, neutrotoxicity seen with vincristine or cisplatin, pulmonary toxicity with a number of different agents but in particular, bleomycin, and steroid toxicity including myopathy, diabetes, hypertension, osteoporosis amongst others. These side-effects and toxicities must be carefully considered and monitored before continuing the use of certain drugs, particularly if there are indications that very early toxicity already exists.

In susceptible tumors, a rapid destruction of bulky tumor masses can produce uric acid nephropathy. To prevent this complication, adequate fluid intake, alkalinization of urine, and administration of allopurinol (300 mg/day by mouth) are indicated during the first period of induction chemotherapy. In some extremely sensitive tumors, a tumor lysis syndrome can occur before or during therapy and dialysis may be required in order to control this complication. Accordingly blood electrolytes and other standard biochemistry values should be monitored during active therapy.

DRUGS: GENERAL PRINCIPLES

Manufacturers supply pharmaceutical information and precautions with each drug and in principal these should be carefully followed. Particular attention should be paid to storage and stability instructions and the recommended methods of administration and dilution. Drugs are usually classified by their *mechanism of action* into three main general categories. Type 1, *non-specific*, i.e. kills cells irrespective of whether the cell is in mitotic cycle or not; type 2, *cell cycle phase-specific*, only kills cells in a particular phase of the mitotic cell cycle; type 3, *non-phase cycle-specific*, only kills cells in mitotic cycle, but in any phase of the cycle. Drugs can also be classified generally into the following major groups: (1) Alkylating agents; (2) antimetabolites, (3) antitumor antibiotics; (4) plant alkaloids; (5) enzymes and random synthetics; (6) hormones; (7) nitrosureas; (8) miscellaneous category.

MECHANISMS OF ACTION: GENERAL COMMENTS

Cytotoxic drugs affect cell divisions and thereby, indirectly, cell proliferation. The different chemotherapeutic agents interfere with a variety of essential cellular events occurring during the process of cell proliferation, e.g. alkylating agents act by the transfer of alkyl groups to cell constituents, such as amino, carboxyl, sulfydryl or phosphate causing impaired function of these important biological cell constituents. Nitrosureas exhibit alkylating agent activity, while enzymes such as L-asparaginase have the unique property of depleting asparagine in tumor cells. Antimetabolites interfere with the synthesis of purine and pyrimidine nucleotides which are the essential building blocks for nucleic acids, while the plant alkaloids produce mitotic arrest by binding to precursors of the spindle. Many of the antitumor antibiotics bind selectively to DNA, forming complexes that block the formation of DNA-dependent RNA.

SIDE-EFFECTS

These may be termed: *immediate* — (acute) occurring during or within 30 minutes of drug administration; *short-term* — within 72 hours of drug administration; *long-term* — after 72 hours some of which may be cumulative and dose-limiting.

The following are most important in assessing the amount of drug to be administered: the performance status of the patient; dose modification when there is myelosuppression or organ dysfunction; evaluation of the objective response of the tumor obtained after therapy and (sub)acute drug toxicity recorded according to the WHO grading scheme.

ANTIEMETICS

The satisfactory control of nausea and vomiting associated with many chemotherapy regimens remains a major challenge to the clinician. It is inappropriate to go into great detail here but in view of the significance of the problem and of recent therapeutic innovations, a brief discussion of the principles of antiemetic therapy is included.

In the last 10 years progress has been made in optimising the use of 'traditional' antiemetics such as phenothiazines (chlorpromazine, prochlorperazine, thiethylperazine), metoclopramide, benzodiazepines (lorazepam) steroids (dexamethasone), and more recently domperidone. Three principles underlie successful treatment:

- combine 2 or more agents with different modes of action e.g. metoclopramide and dexamethasone.
- give adequate doses I.V. of all drugs prior to chemotherapy and, where relevant, continue *regular* dosing during chemotherapy with the aim of prophylaxis rather than treatment of symptoms once they occur.
- after use of the most emetogenic cytotoxic drugs or combinations, continue to give *regular* prophylactic oral antiemetics for 3 to 5 days.

Effective use of antiemetics is best promoted by protocol orientated prescribing agreed by experienced clinicians: it should not be left to the choice of individual junior doctors. Adherence to these principles, however, remains of limited success against symptoms due to drugs such as cisplatin, at doses >50mg/m^2, after which even high dose metoclopramide produces complete control of emesis in only 15–30% of patients.

1990 has seen the launch of the first (ondansetron) of a new generation of antiemetics, the HT3 antagonists, which have been under investigation for this indication since 1986. Under some circumstances (cisplatin >50mg/m^2) ondansetron has been shown to be very effective against acute emesis i.e. within 24 hours of chemotherapy (complete control in 40–50% of patients). It also has the advantage of apparently being almost completely free of significant side-effects. However its efficacy against delayed emesis (>24 hours after chemotherapy) and superiority over established agents for the treatment of symptoms due to less emetogenic chemotherapy remain unproven and it is at present significantly more expensive than the established drugs. Further work is therefore essential to precisely identify the role of the HT3 antagonists in hemato-oncology, to clearly define the most appropriate dose schedules and indications for cost-effective use and therefore to ensure that optimum symptom control is available to as many patients as possible.

Information kindly provided by Timothy Root, Chief Pharmacist, Royal Marsden Hospital, UK.

RECOMMENDED READING

Carter, S.K., Bakowski, M.T. and Hellmann, K. (1987). *Chemotherapy of Cancer,* 3rd edn. New York: Churchill Livingstone.

Cassciato, D.A. and Lowitz, B.B. (1989). *Manual of Clinical Oncology,* 2nd edn. Boston Mass.: Little Brown & Co.

Hellmann, K. and Carter, S.K. (1987). *Fundamentals of Cancer Chemotherapy.* New York: McGraw Hill.

De Vita, V.T., Jr, Hellmann, K. and Rosenberg, S.A. (1989). *Cancer: Principles and Practice of Oncology,* 3rd edn, pp. 1671–1931. Philadelphia: J.B. Lippincott Co.

PART 1

COMMON DRUGS USED IN TREATMENT

RELEVANT CHEMOTHERAPEUTIC AGENTS

ACTINOMYCIN D

Synonyms: Dactinomycin D, [Lyorac Cosmegen]

Mechanism of Action: Cell cycle phase non-specific, but most active in S- and G_1-phases of cell cycle. Intercalates between DNA base pairs and inhibits DNA-dependent RNA synthesis and particularly ribosomal RNA. It has a long half-life, is not metabolized and is excreted mostly in the bile and small amounts in the urine.

Administration: IV

Dosage: 0·015–0·040 mg/kg body weight (1·0–2·5 mg) weekly for 3–5 weeks, at which time bone-marrow depression or gastrointestinal ulceration occurs. Withold drug for 2–4 weeks to allow marrow recovery and repeat course. Another schedule used is 0·015 mg/kg for 5 successive days for a total dose of 0·075 mg/kg. Courses are to be repeated at 2–4 week intervals. Patients with impaired marrow function or recent radiation therapy should have reduced dosages.

Toxicity: ***Local***: Severe pain and local reaction with extravasation. *Ulcerations* will occur, with painful skin necrosis.

Acute: Nausea and vomiting beginning 2 hours after administration. Following repetitive doses it is not unusual for the patient to vomit prior to the medication. Occasionally abdominal pain and diarrhea may occur.

Late: Bone-marrow suppression occurs 3–10 days after the last dose. Dose readjustment should be made if a WBC count is below 3×10^9/l or platelets below 100×10^9/l.

Oral ulcerations, stomatitis, proctitis, diarrhea and abdominal cramps may occur. Lethargy, anorexia, weight loss, unexplained fever, alopecia, erythema, desquamation and hyperpigmentation of skin, especially in areas subjected to irradiation, reversible acneiform eruption, transient serum glutamic oxaloacetic transaminase (SGOT) elevations.

ADRENAL CORTICOSTEROIDS – DEXAMETHASONE, PREDNISONE, PREDNISOLONE

Synonyms: [Meticorten, Deltacortisone, Decadron, Dalalone, Hexadrol, Deltacortril, Oradexon]

Mechanism of Action: Lymphocytolytic but not cytotoxic

Administration: per os (PO), IM, IV

Dosage: *Prednisone:* 10–100 mg/day daily or its prednisolone equivalent, is the commonly employed dosage. In certain protocols the dose used is 40–60 mg/m^2/day.

Dexamethasone: 4–16 mg in daily divided doses. For raised intracranial pressure start with 10 mg IV initially, followed by 4 mg IM or PO, 6 hourly, then taper.
High-dose methylprednisolone is used either alone or with Alkeran or in combination with vincristine and Adriamycin for myeloma, 800 mg/m^2 or 1·5 g for 1–5 days.

Toxicity: ***Acute:*** None

Late: Peptic ulceration, gastrointestinal bleeding, iatrogenic Cushing's syndrome, psychosis, hypertension, osteoporosis, electrolyte imbalance, diabetes and increased susceptibility to infection, particularly herpes zoster and reactivation of tuberculosis.

Hematologic — polycythemia, leucocytosis; muscle weakness due to potassium loss, sodium retention which may result in edema and hypertension, accumulations of fat on the face and trunk, myopathy, loss of skin collagen resulting in thin skin and cutaneous striae, retardation of growth in children, acneiform eruption.

There is minimal sodium-retaining activity with dexamethasone.

Comments and Special Precautions: Patients who will be on chronic corticosteroid administration may have to be placed on prophylactic antituberculous therapy in order to prevent reactivation of latent tuberculosis.

Corticosteroids are extremely useful in hypercalcemia, localized edema secondary to tumor (such as superior vena caval syndrome, spinal cord compression with impending paraplegia) and during radiation therapy to the spinal cord or skull .

Excluding the gastric distress, which can be alleviated with a bland diet, antacids and therapy with ranitidine, the major complication is gastrointestinal bleeding. Occasional instances of lymphoma in the small bowel, responding to corticosteroids, have led to an acute surgical situation, because of perforation. Abdominal perforation can remain asymptomatic in a patient on steroids.

High-dose prednisone will mask fever, which may be the only indication of bacterial or fungal infection.

In patients who have chronic lymphocytic leukemia (CLL), the use of steroids can produce a transient marked increase in the total WBC count, which generally precedes a response.

Euphoria and an increase in appetite is generally produced with corticosteroid therapy and may be extremely useful in the general management of patients with neoplastic disease. However, one should be on guard for more severe psychiatric manifestations which, in the extreme, may lead to personality change, emotional lability and even major psychoses.

AMSACRINE (*m*-AMSA)

Compound: *m*-AMSA (4′ [(9′-acridinyl) amino] methanesulfone-*m*-anisidide)

Synonym: [Amsidine]

Mechanism of action: Cell cycle phase non-specific; all stages of the cell cycle are affected and it has a preferential effect on dividing cells, but particularly in the S-phase.

Administration: IV, over 30–60 min

Dosage: 120–200 mg/m^2 given on days 1–3 as part of combination chemotherapy for induction, or together with high-dose cytosine arabinoside (Ara-C) for a total dose of 600 mg/m^2, divided over 3 days.

Toxicity: ***Acute***: Increased nausea and vomiting.

Late: *Gastrointestinal tract* toxicity with stomatitis and diarrhea in over one-third of the patients; altered liver function tests with grade 2–3 *hepatoxicity*; about half of the patients develop elevated serum alkaline phosphatase, bilirubin and SGOT levels. Very low incidence of cardiac toxicity (1%).

Warning: m-AMSA can only be given with normal serum potassium levels, otherwise life-threatening cardiac arrhythmias can occur. Potassium chloride is infused at the rate of 10 mmol/h during the night before the administraton of *m*-AMSA. Serum electrolytes are evaluated in the morning, to ensure that the serum potassium levels are above 4mmol/l. *m*-AMSA may be given within 4 h of documenting a normal serum potassium level. Serum creatinine and bilirubin levels should be less than 2 mg/dl before *m*-AMSA can be given.

L-ASPARAGINASE

Synonyms: [Elspar]

Mechanism of Action: Cell cycle phase-specific for post-mitotic G_1-phase. Hydrolyzes asparagine into aspartic acid and ammonia and also decreases glutamic acid. These actions result in rapid inhibition of protein synthesis and a delayed inhibition of DNA and RNA synthesis. The plasma half-life ranges from 8 to 30 h, but is constant for each patient. The metabolism of the drug is independent of renal and hepatic function and is not recovered in the urine.

Administration: IV or IM

Dosage: A number of different schedules have been used and a variety of dosages have been given, with predictable toxicity. The most commonly employed schedule is 200 i.u./kg/day IV for 10–28 days, but dosages have varied from 50–2000 i.u./kg/day and weekly or bi-weekly schedules have also been used. In one of the standard protocols used for acute lymphoblastic leukemia (ALL) it is given IV, at 5000 i.u./m^2/day on days 1–14 of the induction regimen. In other schedules the drug has been used at 6000 i.u./m^2 IM twice or thrice weekly starting on day 4, for 3–4 weeks; it has also been used later during induction at 200 i.u./kg/day IM for 15 days.

Toxicity: ***Acute:*** Anaphylatic shock has been described because of hypersensitivity, therefore a small test dose of 2 i.u. is given ID. Epinephrine, hydrocortisone and antihistaminics should be readily available at the bedside to treat acute hypersensitivity if it occurs. Other hypersensitivity reactions may occur with the development of a rash, urticaria, hypotension and moderate respiratory distress with wheezing. Fever, serum-sickness-like syndromes, epigastric pain, nausea and vomiting, lethargy and somnolence may also develop.

If there are any signs of hypersensitization to *Escherichia coli* asparaginase, change to the *Erwinia* asparaginase preparation, performing skin tests before continuing; desensitization may be necessary. If these complications still recur, administration of the drug *must* be stopped.

Anorexia, nausea and vomiting occur in about half of the patients and appear to be dose-dependent. Lethargy, somnolence and confusion can occur in patients receiving increasing doses, which is the main reason for the preference for the lower doses given in recent years.

Late: *Hepatotoxicity* with biochemical evidence of dysfunction in about half of the patients (elevation of serum alkaline phosphatase, bilirubin and SGOT levels). If serum bilirubin levels remain high, dose modification must be introduced.

Hemorrhagic pancreatitis and non-ketotic *hyperglycemia* have been reported in 2–10% of treated patients and are increased when the drug is used with steroids. Acute pancreatitis is an indication for stopping the drug, while hyperglycemia can be treated with insulin without discontinuing therapy.

Coagulation defects vary but generally are subclinical. There are alterations in prothrombin time, partial thromboplastin time and fibrinogen levels with decreased synthesis of clotting factors. Decreased antithrombin 3 levels may also result in thrombotic phenomena but this does not always occur.

Coagulopathy without bleeding or thrombosis is not necessarily an indication to stop the drug but to provide immediate supportive replacement therapy with fresh frozen plasma.

Indeed it is possible that all patients given prolonged courses of asparaginase may have disturbed coagulation, but this may only become a major problem if they also have prolonged thrombocytopenia and sepsis. A keen awareness of this problem may reduce its morbidity and mortality.

Neurological disturbances occur in about half of the patients, including mild depression and personality changes, lethargy, somnolence, impaired sensorium and even coma. EEG changes are not unusual.

Decreased serum cholesterol levels and hypolipidemia are frequent, but hyperlipidemia can also occur. Hypoproteinemia, decreased acute phase reactants and serum complement levels are also frequently seen. Hypocalcemia, due to decrease in the levels of protein-bound calcium occur. The increased blood urea, nitrogen and ammonia levels encountered are due to the action of the drug and not to toxicity.

Bone-marrow suppression occurs in 10–20% of patients.

From recent studies it is clearly evident that *Erwinia* asparaginase has a lower incidence of toxicity than *Escherichia coli* asparaginase, particularly with regard to neurological complications and the incidence of pancreatitis. Anaphylaxis occurs far less frequently using IM *Erwinia*-type asparaginase, and this form of the drug also induces less hepatotoxicity and coagulopathy and is also less diabetogenic.

5-AZACYTIDINE

Mechanism of Action: Cell cycle phase-specific. The drug is an analog of cytidine and is rapidly incorporated into both RNA and DNA, acting as an antimetabolite. The process of translation of nucleic acid sequences is disrupted, thereby inhibiting protein synthesis. It also affects *de novo* pyrimidine synthesis. The drug undergoes rapid hydroloysis and is quickly excreted in the urine within 24 hours.

Administration: IV

Dosage: Usually 150-200 mg/m^2 is given in continuous infusion for 1–5 days. Others have used it at higher doses (300–400 mg/m^2) for 2 days in combination with other drugs, like VP-16.

Toxicity: ***Acute:*** Severe nausea, vomiting and diarrhoea which are dose related and dose-limiting.

Late: *Myelosuppression* occurs regularly with the major nadir occurring at 15–25 days. *Hepatoxicity* after 3–4 weeks. *Rare neurological* effects.

BLEOMYCIN

Synonym: [Blenoxane]

Mechanism of Action: Cytotoxic antibiotic; cell cycle phase-specific with cell division arrested in G_2 specifically. It can also be active in the G_1-, early S- and M-phases. The drug inhibits DNA-synthesis, produces fission of single-stranded DNA, and inhibits cell DNA ligase. The drug is rapidly distributed throughout the body but concentrates in the skin, lung and kidneys, but is not inactivated in skin and lung. Excreted mostly in the urine.

Administration: IV, IM, SC or intracavitary (IC)

Dosages: Different schedules have been used and the drug can be given on its own for successive days, continuously or intermittently as part of other combination chemotherapy regimens. Some regimens use it at 4 mg/m^2 IV on day 1, others (MACOP-B) 10 mg/m^2 IV every 4 weeks or even 15 mg IV on day 14 (COPBLAM). In the newer COPBLAM regimen it is given on day 1 as a 7·5 mg/m^2 IV push followed by a continuous infusion on days 2–5, in order to minimize toxicity.

Bleomycin can also be given at 2·5–5 mg/m^2 IV on 3 successive days every 4–6 weeks. It has also been given as self-administered SC in a dose range of 0·5–1 mg.

When given IC after initial drainage, 60 units is injected into the drainage cannula after being dissolved in 100 ml of normal saline. In pleural effusions withdraw the drug after 24 h.

Toxicity: The highest concentrations of the drug are found in the lung, skin and kidney and in the first two sites the drug is not rapidly inactivated. Bleomycin is excreted in the urine, mostly as an active compound, and accordingly it should be used with caution in patients with renal or pulmonary disease

Acute: Following injection, fever and chills are frequent, as is nausea and vomiting. Anorexia is rare.

In some cases the first doses are accompanied by hyperpyrexia and hypotension with cardiorespiratory collapse, but this is rare. Skin tests are recommended.

Late: In many of the earlier regimens pulmonary complications were encountered. Serious toxicity (fibrosis) occurred in only about 10%. The usual sequence is to have mild to moderate pulmonary toxicity, starting after the 3rd to 4th cycle of treatment. ARDS-type syndrome can occur.

Toxicity is generally related to the total dose administered and 300 mg is the limit to be used. Pulmonary function tests appear to be of no predictive value and patients may present unpredictably with dyspnea. Differential diagnosis is difficult and secondary fungal pneumonia, toxoplasmosis or pneumocystis carinii must be excluded. If chest X-ray or lung function abnormalities are evident, the drug must be stopped immediately and bronchoscopy or lung biopsy may have to be performed in order to finalize the diagnosis. High-dose prednisone (60–100 mg/day) has resulted in reversal of this clincial syndrome.

Alopecia is dose-dependent and occurs frequently. Hyperpigmentation, nail and skin changes with pruritic erythema, nail ridging, hardening of the finger tips, and bulla formation in the skin occur, especially in areas of pressure or irritation.

BUSULFAN

Synonym: [Myleran]

Mechanism of Action: Alkylating agent. Cell cycle phase non-specific. Transfers alkyl groups to important cell constituents including phosphate, sulfhydryl, amido or cortoxyl groups, causing impaired function. DNA guanine is altered and an abnormal base pair is formed with thymidine. It can also cleave the imidazole ring, destroying guanine or alternatively cross-link DNA strands interfering with replication. DNA strand breakage also occurs due to DNA depurination. The drug is well absorbed following oral administration, disappears from the blood quickly and is mostly excreted in the urine.

Administration: PO

Dosage: 2–8 mg daily to approximate total doses of 150–250 mg, then readjust the dose for maintenance therapy according to the bone-marrow status and WBC or platelet counts. The usual maintenance dose is 1–3 mg/day. The drug may be given continuously or intermittently.

Recently high-dose busulfan has been used as bolus therapy prior to bone-marrow transplantation either alone or more frequently with high doses of cyclophosphamide. The commonly used high dose is 16 mg/kg in four divided doses, i.e. 3·5–4·0 mg/kg/day for 4 days, with cyclophosphamide, (60 mg/kg/day) for 2 days.

Toxicity: ***Acute:*** rarely nausea, gastrointestinal dysfunction, alopecia.

Late: Myelosuppression which is dose-limiting because thrombocytopenia, anemia and particularly leukopenia continue for 2–3 weeks after discontinuation of the drug. Bone-marrow aplasia and fibrosis can occur. Careful attention must be paid to the blood counts during therapy and it is recommended that Busulfan be stopped when the WBC reaches 15×10^9/l.

An Addisonian-like syndrome is frequently seen with skin hyperpigmentation, due to an increase in melanin-producing hormone. Gynecomastia is occasionally seen with amenorrhea or testicular atrophy.

Cytologic dysplasia has been found in the uterine cervix, lung and other epithelial tissues. The drug may be terratogenic with the production of fetal malformation, including lens changes and rare cataract formation occurring as ocular toxicity.

Rare but selective pulmonary insufficiency with persistent cough, progressive dyspnea and interstitial pulmonary fibrosis may occur.

CARBOPLATIN

Synonyms: Cis-dichloro cyclobutane dicarboxylato platinum, [Paraplatin, CBDCA, JM-8]

Mechanism of Action: Cell cycle, phase-non-specific but the G_1-phase is most sensitive. Inhibits DNA synthesis. Complementary strands of DNA are cross-linked, with guanine as the preferred binding site. Thus there is inter- and intra-strand alkylation and rival depression. The drug is rapidly cleared from the plasma via the kidneys and as much as 70% is recovered in the urine within the first day.

Administration: IV

Dosages: 200–400 mg/m^2 IV every 4 weeks. Lower doses should be used in previously treated patients or in those with impaired renal function.

Toxicity: ***Acute:*** Rare allergies, anaphylaxis, nausea and vomiting occur but are rarely severe.

Late: Myelosuppression – dose-limiting toxicity, dependent on initial renal function. Leukopenia and thrombocytopenia, nadir at 14–25 days; anemia is cumulative.

Nausea and vomiting can occur as late as 6 h after IV administration and may sometimes persist.

Renal function is rarely affected, but it is important in relation to the eventual degree of myelosuppression that may develop. Keep a careful check on serum creatinine levels and the creatinine clearance.

Peripheral neuropathy and cytotoxicity have been reported but less than in patients treated with cis-platin.

The high volume pre- or post-hydration is not recommended as for cis-platin.

CARMUSTINE

Synonyms: BCNU, (1,3-bis)(2-chloroethyl)(1-nitrosurea), [BiCNU]

Mechanism of Action: Cell cycle phase non-specific. This nitrosurea has alkylating agent activity, mediated through metabolites which alkylate DNA and interfere with DNA repair and DNA enzymes. Tissue uptake is rapid with quick metabolism, accordingly the drug is not found in the plasma. Carmustine crosses the blood–brain barrier and excretion is mostly renal.

Administration: IV

Dosages: Most frequently given at 3–5 mg/kg (200 mg/m^2 IV every 6 weeks, or 90–100 mg/m^2 IV for 2-3 days, consecutively).

High-dose carmustine may be used as part of the preparatory regimen for autologous bone-marrow transplant (ABMT), given as 450–600 mg/m^2 over 6 h.

Toxicity: ***Local:*** Burning sensation may occur during administration with some facial flushing, which can be avoided by readjusting the infusion rate. The drug can cause severe ulceration and fibrosis on extravasation.

Acute: Severe nausea and vomiting occur within the first 2–3 h and may even last up to 48 h. Facial flushing, and light-headness can also occur initially.

Late: Delayed bone-marrow toxicity is dose-dependent and involves all cell lineages, occuring as late as 5–6 weeks after administration.

Renal dysfunction and hepatoxicity occurs occasionally with elevated blood urea nitrogen (BUN) and altered SGOT levels. Rare interstitial pulmonary toxicity with pulmonary fibrosis, which is cumulative, has been documented.

Optic neuritis is very rarely seen.

CHLORAMBUCIL

Synonym: [Leukeran]

Mechanism of Action: Alkylating agent. Cell cycle phase non-specific (see busulfan). The drug is well absorbed after oral administration and rapidly metabolized to phenylacetic acid mustard, Urinary excretion is low, and little is known about its elimination.

Administration: PO

Dosage: Start with 0·1–0·2 mg/kg for 3–6 weeks. Reduce dosage for maintenance, usually to 2 mg/day, depending on the peripheral blood and bone-marrow response. Other schedules use different doses, intermittently as 'pulse' therapy with or without prednisone, employing 15–25 mg/day for 4–5 days every 3 weeks. British studies have also used chlorambucil cyclically to replace mechlorethamine in the MOPP regimen at 10 mg/m^2 for 14 days. A similar regimen of 10 mg/m^2 for 14 days, given every 4–6 weeks, has also been used for CLL.

Toxicity: ***Acute:*** rare, nausea and vomiting with some abdominal discomfort. If this occurs divide the daily dose into several portions or give it preferably at bedtime.

Late: Myelosuppression which is dose-limiting, occurs, developing more slowly than with busulfan and is rapidly reversible.

2-CHLORODEOXYADENOSINE

Synonym: 2-CdA

Mechanism of Action: An adenosine deaminase (ADA) – resistant purine nucleoside, phosphorylated to a nucleotide, by deoxycytidine kinase. These nucleotides accumulate in the cell, particularly in lymphocytes and prevent cells repairing chromosomal breaks properly. This appears to be the proposed mechanism of action of the drug. There is evidence that 2-CdA is incorporated into the DNA of dividing cells.

When infused intravenously it is cleared rapidly, with an initial clearance half time of about 36 minutes followed by a slower component with a half time of 7 hours.

Administration: IV

Dosages: Used in B-cell neoplasias successfully, particularly in hairy cell leukemia (HCL). Recommended dosage is 0·1 mg/kg/day given as a continuous 7 day infusion. The drug is well tolerated and in HCL one cycle of 7 days appears to be sufficient, otherwise given every 4–5 weeks for 6 cycles. Portable infusion pumps have been used recently. It may also be given IV 5 days per week as a 2 hour infusion varying from 0·14–0·7 mg/kg total weekly dose.

Toxicity: ***Acute:*** none

Late: Myelosuppression is observed in only a minority of cases (20%). Lymphopenia and transient monocytopenia may also be seen. Fever may occur in some cases. There is no significant nausea of vomiting and no alopecia.

CISPLATIN

Synonyms: Cis-platinum diamine dichloride, cis-platinum, CDDP, DDP, [Neoplatin, Platinex, Platinol]

Mechanism of Action: It is a heavy metal compound, the parent of carboplatin. Cell cycle phase non-specific but the G_1-phase is most sensitive. Inhibits DNA synthesis. Complementary strands of DNA are cross-linked, with guanine as the preferred binding site. Thus there is inter- and intra-strand alkylation and rival depression. Platinum is detected in the tissues for a few months after treatment. Mostly excreted in the urine.

Administration: IV

Dosages: 50–120 mg/m^2 every 4 weeks or 20 mg/m^2 IV on days 1–5. Others have used 10–60 mg/m^2 every 3 weeks.

Toxicity: ***Acute:*** Rarely allergic, but anaphylactic reactions do occur. Nausea and vomiting is severe, usually occurring within 1–2 h of the injection, but may last for up to 24 h.

Late: Nausea and vomiting. Anorexia lasting for 1–7 days may occur. Myelosuppression may be severe and counts can take up to 40 days to recover. Cytotoxicity is usually cumulative with a high incidence of loss of hearing and tinnitus. Peripheral neuropathy is usually seen at an accumulative dose and audiometric monitoring should be performed frequently.

Hepatoxicity is uncommon, usually transient with elevated SGOT levels. Renal toxicity is dose-limiting, and cumulative, with tubular damage. Serum BUN, serum creatinine levels and creatinine clearance must be measured before each therapy. Treatment should be delayed if renal function is abnormal.

High-volume pre- and post-treatment hydration is recommendcd. About 1–2 litres of fluids should be given 12 h prior to IV therapy and the hydration programme must be maintained for 24 h after therapy.

CYCLOPHOSPHAMIDE

Synonyms: [Cytoxan, Endoxan, Neosar]

Mechanism of Action: Cell cycle phase non-specific. Alkylating agent which is effective PO and IV; activated by liver microsomal enzymes to form 4-hydroxycyclophosphamide. The drug is inactive until metabolized. Most is excreted in the urine within 48 h as drug metabolites and about a third as active drug. This should be remembered as the likely cause of the possible local effects on the bladder mucosa. The oral drug should be taken well after meals as enzymes found in food may inactivate the drug.

Administration: IV, PO or intrapleural

Dosages: Orally 75–150 mg/m^2 or 1·5–2·5 m g/kg/day can be used, particularly in pretreated patients who have received prior radiotherapy. The IV doses used vary from 350–750 mg/m^2 to 30–40 mg/kg in single or divided doses. Doses as high as 60 mg/kg are used in certain high-grade lymphomas (such as Burkitt's lymphoma) and as part of the cytoreductive regimen for bone-marrow transplant together with total body irradiation. The 60 mg/kg/day IV may be given on 4 separate days prior to transplant and usually prior to radiotherapy. It has also been used recently, at 120 mg/kg, on a single day, infused over 8 h in the same transplant setting together with etoposide (VP/16) and carmustine.

Maintenance therapy varies, but after a large IV loading dose, further drug cannot be given for at least 21–28 days, until the blood counts have recovered. Oral maintenance is given at 50–150 mg/day, depending on the blood counts.

Toxicity: ***Local:*** None

Acute: Nausea and vomiting which are dose-dependent, can persist for 24–72 h, however, they more frequently start about 6 h after the IV administration. A strange taste in the mouth, hot flushes and nasal congestion can also develop.

Late: Nausea, vomiting, anorexia; alopecia develops in at least 25% of patients and is common; skin hyperpigmentation, ridging of nails. Myelosuppression is dose-limiting and relatively less thrombocytopenia is encountered than with other drugs. Amenorrhea or azoospermia are common; Cardiac necrosis is rare but may occur, usually only after very high single IV doses.

Sterile hemorrhagic cystitis with dysuria, frequency of micturition and hemorrhage may occur and are dose-limiting and even life-threatening at times. Eventual urinary bladder fibrosis and even epithelial atypia can be encountered. This complication can be prevented by maintaining a high fluid intake and with the administration of MESNA. Liberal fluid intake for 2 days following IV therapy and during all oral therapy with frequent micturition, may minimize the risk of this complication.

Inappropriate anti-diurectic hormone (ADH) secretion may occur very rarely.

CYTOSINE ARABINOSIDE (Ara-C)

Synonyms: Cytarabine, 1-ß-D-arabinofuranosyl cytosine, [Cytosar, Alexan]

Mechanism of Action: Cell cycle phase-specific for S-phase, blocks cells between G_1 and S. This antimetabolite is phosphorylated to derivatives producing inhibition of DNA synthesis, by blocking conversion of cytidine diphosphate to deoxycytidine diphosphamate. However it appears that the Ara-CTP derivative does not inhibit the tumor cell reductase efficiently, but inhibits DNA polymerase by competitive inhibition of dCTP rather than by inhibition of polymerase synthesis. It is metabolized in the liver rapidly and excreted as an inactive metabolite in the urine.

Administration: IV, IM, SC and intrathecal (IT).

Dosages: Various schedules and methods of injection have been used. In acute leukemia the typical regular dosage schedule is 3 mg/kg IV daily or every 12 h, given together with an anthracycline and in the past with 6-thioguanine (6-TG). 100–200 mg/m^2 may be given for 7 days as a continuous 24 h infusion or every 12 h for 14 doses, followed by a rest period of 21 days to allow for bone-marrow recovery.

Intermediate (IDAC) or high dose (HiDAC) given as an IV bolus can be used in acute leukemia either alone or with other drugs such as M-AMSA, mitoxantrone or etoposide. The dose employed in these schedules varies from 500 mg/m^2 (IDAC) as a 1 h infusion every 12 h for 12 doses to 3 g/m^2 given during 3 h for 6 days (HiDAC) or every 12 h for 3 days (6 doses), with prophylactic eye washing with steroid eyedrops during therapy. In the newer protocols employed for ALL, it is also given but in a cyclic fashion, at a dose of 75 mg/m^2 IV for 4 days, in association with other drugs such as VP-16 or VM-26.

When given by IM or SC injection for the treatment of myelodysplastic syndromes or even acute leukemia a lower dose (LoDAC) of 10–15 mg/m^2 is given once or twice daily for periods up to 42 days or even longer, depending on the response. The drug has also been given in lymphomas and CLL, in combination with other agents such as cyclophosphamide, oncovin and prednisone, at a dose of 25 mg/m^2 every 12 h for 5 days or even at more conventional doses of 2·5–3·0 mg/kg for 1–4 days.

IT Ara-C can be given in a dose of 30 mg/m^2 (about 50 mg) in sterile saline usually together with methotrexate (MTX) in the treatment of meningeal leukemia.

Toxicity:

Acute: Anorexia, vomiting and nausea, which is dose-related, especially if the infusion is too rapid.

Late: The major side-effect is myelosuppression with leukopenia and thrombocytopenia being the most prominent. Megaloblastic change which may be very marked, occurs in the erythroid cell series. The nadir with conventional IV doses is 7–14 days but with the higher dose schedules this may be more than 28 days. LoDAC produces obvious reduction in marrow cellularity but seldom causes aplasia. Severe granulocytopenia causing sepsis and thrombocytopenia resulting in hemorrhage are encountered quite frequently with this schedule.

Hepatic dysfunction occurs but is usually mild and reversible, resulting in elevations in SGOT and alkaline phosphatase levels which are not dose-limiting in most cases.

'Ara-C syndrome' may develop in some patients, characterized by bone pain, myalgia and pyrexia, sometimes accompanied by chest pain, malaise, conjunctivitis and a rash. This occurs 6–12 h after IV infusion, and may be steroid responsive.

Comments and Precautions: Using the higher doses of Ara-C the major toxicity is hematopoietic and one should have all the facilities available for adequate patient support during the periods of severe leukopenia and thrombocytopenia which may well be prolonged. Without these facilities being available, this therapy cannot be given.

Other life-threatening severe complications can occur with HiDAC including severe stomatitis and gastrointestinal mucositis associated with abdominal pain and diarrhea, sloughing of mucosa and secondary infection. Epithelial dysplasia of the gastrointestinal tract mucosa has also been reported in fatal cases. With HiDAC, marked alterations of liver function are seen with impressive elevations of SGOT, alkaline phosphatase and lactate dehydrogenase. Cerebellar symptoms with confusion, somnolence and ataxia have also been recorded after HiDAC.

Because of the above described toxicities and the fact that results may not be better than with the lower doses, HiDAC therapy has been replaced in many centers by the less toxic doses used in the IDAC regimens.

DACARBAZINE

Synonyms: Imidazole carboxamide, 5-(3,3-dimethyl-l-triazeno)-imidazole-4-carboamide, [DTIC]

Mechanism of Action: The drug has some alkylating agent-like activity and is probably a cell cycle non-specific agent which interacts with sulfydryl groups in proteins. It inhibits purine, RNA and protein synthesis markedly and DNA synthesis only moderately. Appears to prolong G_2 *in vivo* and G_1 *in vitro*. The drug undergoes *N*-demethylation in the liver to form derivatives that are eventually converted to amino imidazole carboxamide, and rapidly excreted by the renal tubules.

Administration: IV

Dosages: The most frequent dose used is 250 mg/m^2 IV on days 1–5 every 21–28 days. In other schedules like ABVD both 250 mg/m^2 and 375 mg/m^2 have been used on days 1 and 8 of the cycle.

Others have used it in single doses as high as 800 mg/m^2 every 3–4 weeks. Lower doses are recommended in patients with myelosuppression or impaired renal function.

Toxicity: *Local:* Some patients complain of a burning sensation during IV administration; pain may be decreased during infusion by withdrawing blood into the dacarbazine-containing syringe and injecting the blood–dacarbazine mixture.

Acute: Nausea and vomiting occur in most patients, appear to be dose-dependent and usually start within 3 h of the IV and can last up to 12 h. Anorexia is also frequently seen; occasionally diarrhoea, facial flushing and paresthesiae can also be seen.

Late: Alopecia occurs and an influenza-like syndrome with myalgia, malaise and fever lasting for 7–21 days may develop infrequently in about 2% of patients, about a week after treatment. Hepatotoxicity with altered liver function tests is infrequent. Myelosuppression, which is dose-limiting, is the most frequent toxicity encountered.

DAUNORUBICIN

Synonyms: Daunomycin, rubidomycin, [cerubidin]

Mechanism of Action: Cell cycle phase non-specific but maximal in S-phase. Cytotoxic antibiotic that intercalates between DNA base pairs with inhibition of DNA-dependent RNA synthesis. Rapidly metabolized in the liver and distributed to tissues. Forty percent of the drug is excreted in the bile and 25% in the urine.

Administration: IV

Dosages: This is the most commonly used anthracycline in acute myeloblasatic leukemia (AML), given daily for 3 days, at a dose between 30 and 60 mg/m^2/day, (usually in combination with Ara-C) every 3–4 weeks. In ALL a lower dose is often used, 25 mg/m^2 IV on days 1, 8, 15, 22 as part of many of the different induction regimens:

In acute promyelocytic leukemia (M3-AML), it is

frequently used during the induction period, at 2 mg/kg/day IV for 5–6 days. Total cumulative dose should never exceed 550 mg/m^2.

Toxicity:

Local: Phlebitis and local irritation occur at the site of injection or extravasation.

Acute: Nausea and vomiting is usually moderate but can be severe; red urine (but not hematuria).

Late: Myelosuppression is the major dose-limiting toxicity and the blood counts return to normal usually within 21 days. Counts returning to normal 21 days later.

Stomatitis, diarrhea and alopecia do occur.

Cardiotoxicity: cardiopulmonary symptoms can occur characterized by transient reversible ECG changes with or without arrhythmias. Of major importance is the possible development of congestive cardiac failure which tends to be seen more frequently above the total cumulative dose of 550 mg/m^2. If signs of cardiac failure occur, discontinue the drug immediately. However, the total dose should never exceed 550 mg/m^2 and patients receiving the drug on a long-term basis should always be monitored for ECG abnormalities and signs of cardiac failure.

Caution: Reduce the dose in patients with impaired hepatic function and avoid giving it to patients with a significant history of cardiac disease.

DEOXYCOFORMYCIN

Synonyms: DCF, [Pentostatin]

Mechanism of Action: Inhibitor of the adenosine deaminase enzyme resulting in accumulation of dATP, and subsequent depletion of nicotinamide adenine dinucleotide and the ATP pool. This induces double-stranded DNA breaks. The drug has a short half-life and is predominantly eliminated in the urine.

Administration: IV

Dosages: Used mostly in hairy cell leukemia but also in various T-cell lymphomas and refractory CLL. The usual regimen is 4 mg/m^2 IV given weekly or every 2 weeks, depending on the counts, for the first 4 injections, followed by monthly injections for the next 4 doses. A total of about 15–16 injections are usually sufficient to obtain a clinical response, but some patients may require more. If the disease remains stable it may be possible to stop therapy after 6 months.

Comment: The drug was used in the past for the treatment of childhood T-ALL using much higher doses. Marked toxicity was encountered at this dose with severe central nervous system symptoms, hepatic, renal and respiratory complications. Because of this, such high doses are no longer used and the drug is not used for ALL therapy at all.

Toxicity: ***Acute:*** Nausea, vomiting and lethargy may be severe.

Late: Elevation in serum creatinine levels. Moderate myelosuppression with neutropenia and lymphopenia can occur resulting in subsequent sepsis in a small proportion of cases.

DOXORUBICIN

Synonyms: Hydroxydaunomycin hydrochloride, [Adriamycin]

Mechanism of Action: Anthracycline antibiotic derivative. Cell cycle phase non-specific, active in all phases of the cycle but mostly in S-phase. Inhibits DNA-dependent RNA synthesis as well as DNA-dependent DNA synthesis mainly by inhibition of topoisomerase II; it also undergoes intercalation between DNA base pairs causing template disorder and steric obstruction.

Rapidly metabolized initially in the blood to a therapeutically active derivative which is also distributed in the liver, heart and kidneys within half a minute. Only 5–10% of the drug is excreted in the urine and most of it is eliminated in the bile.

Administration: IV

Dosages: A variety of schedules have been tried but an acute dosage schedule like in ABV(D) or PROMACE includes 25 mg/m^2 IV given twice during the cycle or 40–50 mg/m^2 given every 3 weeks (as in M-BACOD, MACOP-B or COPBLAM). In ALL, 40–50 mg/m^2 is used every three weeks in the older protocols, while the newer regimens include it at 20–25 mg/m^2 IV given weekly or even more frequently as part of consolidation therapy. In myeloma it is used (in VAD or VAMP) at 9 mg/m^2 as a continuous infusion over 24 h, during days 1–4.

In CLL it has also been used by some at lower IV doses, 15 mg/m^2 on days 1, 8 and 15 of a monthly cycle (POACH), while others have used it at either 25 or 50 mg/m^2 on day 1 of a monthly cycle combined with other drugs (CHOP or CAP).

Toxicity: ***Local:*** Vesicant action with local tissue necrosis; ulceration and phlebitis will occur on extravasation.

Acute: Mild nausea and vomiting is usual; diarrhea, red urine (not hematuria) can occur, while pyrexia is rare.

Late: Rarely, persistent nausea and vomiting occurs. Stomatitis is less common but alopecia develops in most patients. Increased pigmentation in the palms of the hands or soles of the feet and proximal nail beds can be seen and radiosensitization may occur if it is given concomitantly with radiotherapy.

Myelosuppression is the major dose-limiting toxicity and leukopenia is the more significant.

Cardiotoxicity: Transient ECG changes occur in 5–30% of patients including voltage reduction, supraventricular tachyarrhythmias, ventricular premature beats and ST-T wave changes. These occur in the first few days following infusion with very little significant morbidity or mortality. Patients receving more than 550 mg/m^2 have a one in three chance of developing severe, usually irreversible congestive cardiac failure due to a diffuse cardiomyopathy. The latter apparently, has no relationship with pre-existing cardiac disease. Dilation of the heart occurs in this complication and echocardiography and cardiac scans should always be performed repeatedly during therapy to monitor the ejection fraction and cardiac function. There is some evidence to show that concomitant radiotherapy or treatment with cyclophosphamide may potentiate Adriamycin cardiotoxicity, which can occur as late as 6 months after treatment. In this situation the total dose should be limited to 450 mg/m^2.

EPIRUBICIN

Synonyms: [Pharmorubicin, Farmorubicin]

Mechanism of Action: This is a sugar-modified analog of doxorubicin and a 4 epi-analog with inversion of the stereochemistry at the C-4 on the sugar moiety. It is a cell cycle phase non-specific anthracycline; active in all phases of the cell cycle but maximal in S-phase (see doxorubicin). The drug is eliminated primarily in the hepatobiliary system and about 10% is eliminated in the urine.

Administration: IV

Dosages: The usual dose alone is 75–90 mg/m^2 IV. In combination regimens, 50 mg/m^2 is usually given every 3 weeks.

Toxicity: ***Local:*** It is an irritant and vesicant and extravasation: facial flushing may occur sometimes; some nausea and vomiting.

Immediate: Facial flushing may occur. Sometimes nausea and vomiting.

Acute: Nausea and vomiting: diarrhea, red urine (not hematuria) may also be seen.

Late: Alopecia, stomatitis, and nail pigmentation

are seen. Myelosuppression is the major dose-limiting toxicity.

Cardiotoxicity: is less frequently encountered than with doxorubicin, possibly because of the higher plasma clearance. Congestive failure and/or cardiomyopathy may occur when the cumulative dose is more than 900–1000 mg/m^2; and this may be encountered several weeks after discontinuation of therapy. In patients who receive prior anthracyclines, echocardiogram or MUGA cardiac scan should be performed prior to administration of the drug.

ETOPOSIDE

Synonyms: VP-1623, [Vepesid]

Mechanism of Action: This is a semisynthetic podophyllotoxin, causing inhibition of metaphases, thereby preventing cells from entering into mitosis. It is partially cell cycle phase-specific, being active mostly in the S-phase but there is probably some activity in the G_2-phase as well. The drug is excreted in the urine and biliary tract almost equally.

Administration: PO or IV

Dosages: Only 50% of the dose is absorbed orally. The PO dose is 100–300 mg/m^2 daily for 5 days. The IV dose is 60–120 mg/m^2 daily for 5 days or 200 mg/m^2 on days 1–3, given cyclically every 3–4 weeks. It may also be given as part of a high-dose ablative regimen in an higher dose of 1500–2000 mg/m^2, as a continuous infusion over 24 h.

Toxicity: ***Immediate:*** Orthostatic hypotension if given too quickly. Anaphylactic-like reactions are rare.

Acute: Nausea and vomiting occurs.

Late: Myelosuppression occurs and particularly leukopenia and thrombocytopenia. Alopecia is seen in 10–20% of patients. Oral mucosal ulcerations may occur.

FLUDARABINE PHOSPHATE

Synonyms: FAMP, 2-fluoro-ara-AMP.

This is a 2-fluoro 5′-monophosphate derivative of the antileukemic agent 9-Beta-D-arabinofuranosyl adenine arabinoside (Ara-A). This is a novel purine nucleotide analog which is soluble in water and resists deamination by adenosine deaminase.

Mechanism of Action: FAMP is dephosphorylated to 2-fluoro-ara-A and then rephosphorylated intracellulary to 2 fluoro-ara-ATP, the active agent, which curtails DNA synthesis and inhibits ribonucleotide reductase and DNA polymerase alpha. Elimination of the drug is biphasic and the major metabolite in the plasma, 2-FLAA, is deaminated further and is apparently excreted mostly by the kidney.

Administration: IV

Dosage: 20–25 mg/m^2, given as a rapid infusion each day for 5 days, every 28 days.

Toxicity: Myelosuppression with neutropenia and thrombocytopenia in at least a third of the patients; if the neutropenia is severe, there is a tendency to infection, particularly pneumonia. Transient episodes of somnolence, fatigue, nausea and vomiting occur (in about 20% of cases). Isolated cases of pancreatitis, chest pain, pruritus and skin rash have been seen. Blurred vision and peripheral neuropathy are seen in about 10% of patients as is pulmonary toxicity with dyspnea and cough. Stomatitis is seen in a few cases while diarrhea is rare.

If the platelets drop to below $50 \times 10^9/l$, only 15 mg/m^2 is given in the following course.

5-FLUOROURACIL

Synonym: 5-FU

Mechanism of Action: Antimetabolite, S-phase specific. The drug is activated to deoxynucleotide (DN) and catabolized after reduction. Most of it is excreted as respiratory CO_2 and about 10% in the urine.

DN has an affinity for the thymidylate synthetase system, thereby blocking thymidylate synthesis and eventual thymine, pyrimidine bases and DNA synthesis.

Administration: IV, PO, IC and even topical.

Dosage: 12–15 mg/kg for 3 to 5 consecutive days, IV every 4 weeks. In older schedules this was followed by 7·5 mg/kg every other day.

15 mg/kg (maximum 1 g may also be given IV, weekly for 4–6 weeks.

Toxicity: ***Local:*** None

Acute: Nausea, vomiting and anorexia, which is dose-dependent, may occur.

Late: Gastrointestinal complications are common with mucositis, stomatitis, diarrhea and gastroenteritis. The latter may be severe with sloughing and bleeding and can even be fatal. Severe stomatitis is an indication to stop therapy.

Myelosuppression is dose-limiting and leukopenia is more frequent than thrombocytopenia but less frequent when the drug is given as a weekly schedule.

Dermatitis, erythema, nail changes, hyperpigmentation and alopecia can also be seen.

Cerebellar ataxia is uncommon but reversible.

HYDROXYUREA

Synonym: [Hydrea]

Mechanism of Action: Antimetabolite, S-phase-specific but it is possible that the drug also arrests cells in the G_1-phase of the cycle. It inhibits DNA synthesis through inhibition of ribonucleotide reductase, an enzyme that catalyzes conversion of ribonucleotides to deoxyribonucleotides, a crucial step in DNA synthesis. Hydroxyurea is rapidly absorbed from the gastrointestinal tract. Some of the oral dose is metabolized in the liver and then completely cleared in the urine. The drug crosses the blood–barrier.

Administration: PO

Dosage: 60–80 mg/kg PO as a single dose for 3 days and thereafter 20–30 mg/kg/day as a maintenance dose. If there is impaired bone-marrow or renal function it may be used at a dose of 1·5 g twice weekly. An especially high dose of 20 g over 24 h, may also be given.

Toxicity: ***Acute:*** Drowsiness and nausea are rare.

Late: Nausea and vomiting, may be severe. Macopapular rash and alopecia are rare. Myelosuppression is dose-limiting but there is a very quick recovery after discontinuing the drug.

Megaloblastosis and anemia occur but are rare. Stomatitis and renal tubular function impairment occur but are rare and transient.

IDARUBICIN

Synonym: [Zavedos]

This drug is 4-demethoxydaunorubicin. A new analog of doxorubicin, in which a proton replaces the methoxy group in the 4 position, giving the drug enhanced lipophilicity manifested by enhanced penetration through organ and cellular membranes.

Mechanism of Action: The drug is cell cycle phase non-specific but maximal in the S and M phases; like daunorubicin, but inhibits RNA synthesis more potently than daunorubicin. It is however, significantly less cardiotoxic than daunorubicin or doxorubicin. As with other anthracyclines the mechanism of action includes DNA scission (probably attributable to inhibition of topoisomerase II), free radical generation and cell membrane interactions.

Administration: IV or, experimentally, oral.

Dosage: 10–12 mg/m^2/day IV for 3 days every 3 weeks. Oral doses can be 15–20 mg/m^2 or given as 50 mg/m^2 in 4 divided doses on days 1 and 14, though this route is not yet reliably developed.

Toxicity: ***Immediate:*** Mild nausea and vomiting can occur.

Late: Alopecia is most frequent; nausea, diarrhoea and stomatitis usually develop.

A potent bone marrow suppressant. Transient hepatotoxicity occurs with elevations of SGOT and serum bilirubin levels. Reversible ECG changes can occur (T-wave inversion, S-T depression) and transient arrhythmias are rare.

IFOSFAMIDE

Synonyms: [Mitoxana, Holoxan]

Mechanism of Action: The drug is cell cycle phase non-specific; and a structural analog of cyclophosphamide. It is activated by liver microsomal enzymes to 4-hydroxyifosfamide and then excreted by the kidney. It acts as an alkylating agent transferring alkyl groups to important cell constituents as does cyclophosphamide and mechlorethamine.

Administration: IV in a fast-running infusion over 30–120 min or as a continuous infusion over 24 h.

Dosage: 1·0–2·0 g/m^2/day IV, usually for 5 days, every 3-4 weeks.

Higher doses of 5·0–6·0 g/m^2 as an IV infusion over 24 h may be given every 3–4 weeks. If there is impaired renal function, lower doses should be given.

Toxicity: ***Acute:*** Dose-limiting hematuria or 'cystitis' with frequency of micturition or dysuria may occur which can be prevented with MESNA. The patient must be well-hydrated prior to and during therapy. Nausea, vomiting, lethargy and confusion may also occur.

Late: Alopecia occurs, as does myelosuppression; particularly leukopenia which may be dose-limiting. Anemia is less frequent, and thrombocytopenia is rare. Late urinary complications may also occur.

INTERFERON

Synonyms: IFN, [Intron-A, Roferon, Wellferon]

Mechanism of Action: The interferons are a large group of inducible proteins (biological response modifiers) with potent antiviral, antitumor and immunomodulating activities which are classified according to antigenic specificities into three broad classes: the leukocyte-derived alpha-interferon, fibroblast-derived beta-interferon, and T-lymphocyte-produced gamma-interferon. The mechanism(s) of action are unknown but the demonstrable antitumor effect has been putatively attributed to three basic mechanisms: direct antiproliferative effects on tumor cells; induction of a differentiation phenotype in the tumor cells and activation of non-specific host defence mechanisms, such as natural killer cells or macrophage tumoricidal properties.

Cell cycle analysis has shown that interferon causes extension of all phases of the cell cycle and prolongation of the overall cell generation time. In some cases an accumulation of cells in G_0 has been observed, accompanied by a decrease in transition to G_1. The critical mechanisms operative at the cellular level may be mediated by inhibitors of DNA and RNA synthesis. Specifically, induction of 2′-5′ oligoadenylate synthetase (AS) leads to the formation from ATP of 2′-5′-linked oligonucleotides of adenosine. These oligonucleotides activate an endogenous cellular endoribonuclease which degrades both messenger and ribosomal RNA. In addition, a protein kinase and a phosphodiesterase pathway represent mechanisms of inhibition of protein synthesis which are parallel to, but independent of 2′-5′ AS. Whether these are in fact central to antiproliferative activity has not been definitely established. However, elevated levels of 2′-5′AS have been correlated with tumor response in some patients.

Administration: SC or IM

Dosage: Various schedules have been used.

For lymphocytic lymphomas, leukemia, hairy cell leukemia and myeloma, 3×10^6 units/m^2/day every day or 3–5 times per week for a few months is an acceptable dose. If there is response to therapy it appears that interferon has to be continued as maintenance for much more than a year. For chronic myeloid leukemia (ML) larger doses have been used, ranging from 3 to 9×10^6 units/m^2/day for up to a year's duration. It seems now that human α-interferon may best be used in combination with other chemotherapeutic agents including busulfan and hydroxyurea for CGL, chlorambucil prednisone and other more aggressive combination regimens for lymphoma and myeloma and in sequence with deoxycoformycin in hairy cell leukemia.

Toxicity: *Possible adverse events during interferon treatment*

Flu-like symptoms, including fever, chills or rigors, headache, myalgia, lumbar pain, joint pain, paresthesiae/dysaesthesiae, fatigue, abnormal taste in the mouth, anorexia, nausea, hyper-/hypotension, arrhythmia, impairment of consciousness, alopecia.

Because of the potential cardiotoxicity which is rarely encountered, the compound should not be given to elderly patients with a previous history of cardiac disease.

INTERLEUKIN-2 (IL-2)

Mechanism of Action: A biological response modifier, which is a major T-cell growth factor which activates natural killer cells, T-lymphocytes, lymphokine-activated killer (LAK) cells to antitumor activity. Recombinant IL-2 causes a massive expansion of cells with cytotoxic function and may be used alone or in conjunction with the adoptive transfer of LAK cells or tumor-infiltrating lymphocytes (TIL), α-interferon or tumor necrosis factor (TNF).

Administration: IV, SC

Dosage: Different schedules are used.

Continuous dose: $3\text{–}5 \times 10^6$ units/m^2 to maximum tolerance dose for 5 days each week for 4 weeks sometimes with α-interferon ($3\text{–}5 \times 10^6$ units/m^2), intermittent low dose cyclophosphamide or with low dose (70 μg) TNF for 3 days.

High dose: 1×10^6 units/kg IV every 8 h in 50 ml 0·9% saline with 5% albumin until dose-limiting toxicity is reached, usually after 5–6 days. This dose has mostly been given with LAK or TIL cells after an initial injection of cyclophosphamide (25 mg/kg). The TIL are given as 2×10^{11} cells in 200–250 ml infusions over a period of 30–60 min. These doses are seldom used conventionally.

Toxicity: Side-effects relate to an increased vascular permeability, leading to loss of intravascular volume and accumulation of fluids in the soft tissues and visceral organs. Thus 25% of patients gain weight which resolves after discontinuation of IL-2. More side-effects are also encountered when *LAK cells* are given with IL-2. Chills, fever, rigors in almost all the patients; nausea, vomiting, diarrhea in almost half the patients; hypotension in over 70%, erythema and pruritus, fatigue, lethargy, mental confusion, disorientation, oliguria, increased creatinine levels, acute renal failure, respiratory distress, hyperbilirubinemia. All the above are dose-limiting and will be less severe and less frequent in protocols not employing LAK cells and at lower doses of IL-2 infusion.

LOMUSTINE

Synonyms: CCNU (1-(2-chloroethyl)-3-cyclohexyl-l-nitrosurea), [CEENU]

Mechanism of Action: Alkylating-agent-like activity, cell cycle phase non-specific agent. The chloroethyl isocyanate portion of the molecule results in carbamylation of amino acids and proteins. The drug acts as an alkylating agent but also appears to inhibit several key enzymes involved in DNA synthesis. The drug is rapidly metabolized and 50% is excreted in the urine within 12 h. It crosses the blood–brain barrier.

Administration: PO

Dosage: Various schedules have been used. 100–130 mg/m^2 PO as a single dose used every 6 weeks is the recommended dose if there is no marrow impairment. For pre-existent marrow depression lower doses (50–100 mg/m^2) are used.

Toxicity: ***Immediate:*** None

Acute: Nausea and vomiting 4–6 h after use, persisting for up to 2 days.

Late: Nausea, vomiting, stomatitis, is uncommon; rarely alopecia, reversible altered liver function tests, cumulative myelosuppression, with more thrombocytopenia than leucopenia.

MECHLORETHAMINE

Synonyms: Nitrogen mustard, Mustine, [Mustargen]

Mechanism of Action: Alkylating agent, cycle non-phase-specific but most active in the M- and G_1-phases of the cell cycle. Acts by the transfer of alkyl groups to important constituents such as amino, carboxyl, sulfhydryl or phosphate groups causing their impaired function. Alkylation of guanine in the DNA leads to the formation of an abnormal base pair with thymidine, partial destruction of guanine, cross-linkage of DNA strands preventing replication and eventual breakage of DNA strands. The compound is rapidly hydrolyzed, cleared quickly from the blood and excreted mostly in the urine.

Administration: IV, IC

Dosage: 10 mg/m^2 or even 16 mg/m^2 (0·4 mg/Kg) IV as a single dose. May also be divided during 2–4 consecutive days, given through a running IV infusion. Typical doses in MOPP regimen, 6 mg/m^2 IV doses on days 1 and 8.

Can be given IC after reconstitution in 100–200 ml of normal saline. Inject the dose equivalent of the IV dose and quickly move the patient from the prone to a supine position in order to distribute the drug.

Toxicity: ***Local:*** The drug is a vesicant and if spillage takes place local desquamation and ulceration occurs, special care must be taken when veins with previous thrombosis are used for IV infusion. Venous fibrosis occurs. Be careful to protect eyes and skin when the drug is being mixed and administered.

Acute: Severe nausea and vomiting lasting for several hours; chills and rigors; Metallic taste in the mouth, anti-emetic agents and sedatives (100 mg phenobarbitone or seconal PO and a phenothiazine) are invariably needed when this drug is given and may have to be repeated.

Late: Myelosuppression, mostly leukopenia occurring about 15 days after therapy. This is usually dose-limiting. Thrombocytopenia also occurs.

Temporary or permanent oligo-amenorrhea occurs in females while decreased spermatogenesis and azoospermia develops in males, which is associated with temporary and quite frequently with permanent sterility.

MELPHALAN

Synonyms: L-phenylalanine mustard (L-PAM), L-Sarcolysin, [Alkeran]

Mechanism of Action: Alkylating agent (mechlorethamine). Class 3, cell cycle non-specific. The drug is a phenylalanine derivative of mechlorethamine and is well absorbed when given PO or IV. Remains active in the blood for about 6 h, It is excreted in the urine and if renal function is impaired reduced dosages may be needed.

Administration: PO or IV

Dosage: One schedule employs a loading dose initially, 0·25 mg/kg/day for 4 days, followed by 0·1–0·15 mg/kg/day for 7–10 days followed by no therapy for 2–4 weeks depending on the blood counts. Alternatively, therapy can begin at 2–6 mg/day with adjustments made depending on the blood counts. Intermittent or continuous treatment can be given. Reduce the dosage or stop the drug if renal function is impaired, depending on how bad the glomerular filtration is.

A high-dose schedule is also used in patients with responsive myeloma who will be treated with bone-marrow autografting. Up to 200 mg/m^2 may be given, while 90–140 mg/m^2 may be given if subsequent autografting is not performed.

Toxicity: ***Immediate:*** Nausea, vomiting is rare but may occur with high doses.

Acute: Oral mucosal ulceration.

Late: Myelosuppression, most frequently leukopenia and thrombocytopenia which is often delayed and may persist for weeks or even months. Amenorrhea and infertility is seen. Alopecia is rare.

6-MERCAPTOPURINE

Synonyms: 6-MP, [Purinethol]

Mechanism of Action: Antimetabolite, cell cycle S-phase-specific which is converted intracellularly to 6-thioinosinic acid, a ribonucleotide which can suppress *de novo* purine biosynthesis and has other effects on purine metabolism. It is inactivated in the liver through oxidation via xanthine oxidase, and excreted in the urine.

Administration: PO

Dosage: 2–5 mg/kg/day or 60 mg/m^2/day

Toxicity: ***Immediate:*** none

Acute: nausea, vomiting

Late: Anorexia, stomatitis and diarrhea are rare. Cholestatic hepatic dysfunction occurs in a third of the patients, which is usually reversible. Myelosuppression which occurs may last for several days after cessation of the drug. Leukopenia is particularly common.

Caution: If allopurinol is given concomitantly, the dose should be reduced to a third, because 6-MP is primarily metabolized by xanthine oxidase, which is blocked by allopurinol.

METHOTREXATE (MTX)

Synonym: Amethopterin

Mechanism of Action: Antimetabolite and folic acid antagonist which is cell cycle S-phase-specific. It acts by almost irreversible binding to dihydrofolate reductase, an enzyme that reduces folic acid to tetrahydrofolic acid, thereby resulting in depletion of tetrahydrofolate which is so vital for the biosynthesis of thymidylic acid (DNA) and inosinic acid (part of RNA synthesis). Leukemic cells have an increased nucleic acid synthesis and are thus more affected by the action of MTX, than normal cells. This block in dihydrofolate reduction can be bypassed by the use of leucovorin (also known as (citrovorum factor or folinic acid). MTX is readily absorbed from the gastrointestinal tract and peaks 0·5–2 h after IV administration. It is widely distributed in body tissues with the highest concentrations in the kidney, gall bladder, liver and skin. Most of the drug is excreted unchanged in the urine within 24 h, after most of it is eliminated by glomerular filtration and active tubular transport. Repeated doses may lead to plasma and tissue accumulation. Retention in body fluids increases toxicity and renal function impairment also increases serum and tissue level of the drug.

Administration: IV, IM, IT and PO

Dosage: Many dosage schedules have been employed. Orally 1·25–2·5 mg daily or as a weekly maintenance dose for ALL has been used in young children; alternatively 20–30 mg/m^2 once to twice weekly has been used more frequently and this may be adjusted later according to the toxicity or response.

Older children or adults may receive 5–10 mg daily (3–4 × the child dosage) for a limited time period, once again adjusting the dose according to the hematologic status.

In lymphoma, particularly high-grade lymphoma, much higher doses have been employed varying from regimen to regimen. Some initial schedules employed what would today be considered as a relatively low dose of 30–60 mg/m^2 per week every 3–4 weeks. Other protocols (m-BACOD) used intermediate doses, 200–500 mg/m^2 IV on days 1 and 8 of a 21–28 day cycle followed by leucovorin rescue (10 mg/m^2 every 6 h for 6 doses starting 24 h after MTX.

In the MACOP-B regimen, 400 mg/m^2 IV every 3–4 weeks is used in which 100 mg/m^2 is given over the first hour as an IV bolus, followed by 300 mg/m^2 IV infusion over 4 h with leucovorin rescue (15 mg, orally every 6 h for 6 doses, 24 h after completion of MTX therapy).

In the PROMACE combination it is used at a higher dose 1500 mg/m^2, over 12 h, on day 14 of a 28-day cycle, followed by 50 mg/m^2 leucovorin IV rescue, every 6 h for 5 doses, starting 24 h after MTX completion.

In other protocols for undifferentiated or lymphoblastic lymphoma it is given at 300 mg/m^2 over the first hour as a bolus, followed by 60 mg/m^2 between hours 2–42 (total dose of 2700 mg/m^2) with leucovorin rescue.

In the M-BACOD regimen, prior to m-BACOD, it was initially used at a much higher dose, 3·0-7·5 g/m^2, IV on day 14 of a 28-day cycle followed by leucovorin rescue every 3 h and then every 6 h for 72 h (12 mg/m^2 IV). One example of the procedure and schedules used for very high doses IV MTX with leucovorin is now described.

HIGH-DOSE MTX DETAILS OF A REGIMEN

1. High-dose MTX should always be given in hospital. Patients are hospitalized the evening before MTX infusion and discharged 48–72 h later, providing no complications occur.

2. Dose and schedule of MTX administration:
   (a) Adequate hydration (3 litres of fluid per day) either PO or IV for at least 48 h following MTX.
   (b) Urine alkalinization aimed at continually maintaining a pH above 7, must start the night before MTX infusion by the administration of 3 g sodium bicarbonate, PO every 3 h and continued for 48 h (either PO or IV) following MTX infusion. All urine samples are checked for pH and if they fall below 7 additional bicarbonate must be given.
   (c) The initital dose of MTX is 1 g/m^2, given as an IV infusion over 6 h.
   (d) Dosage escalation. In the absence of significant toxicity, doses are escalated every 2 weeks to 1·5 g/m^2, 3g/m^2, 6 g/m^2, and three weeks later to 7·5 g/m^2. Once it is reached it is repeated every 3 weeks. Dosage escalation is not continued if a patient develops MTX toxicity such as stomatitis, nephrotoxicity (increase in serum

creatinine over 50% of baseline value) and myelosuppression with a total granulocyte count below $0{\cdot}5\times10^9$/l, despite adequate leucovorin rescue. Patients are to receive subsequent courses at the highest dosage which was not associated with significant toxicity at 3 week intervals.

(e) Serum MTX levels must be measured immediately at cessation of MTX infusion and 24, 48, 72 h after infusion. Further measurements are done as indicated by baseline values and the clinical course.

(f) Serum creatinine levels must be obtained 24 and 48 h after MTX infusion. If at 24 h it is 50% or more above the baseline value, IV fluids must be increased and the serum level repeated at 36 h. If it is still elevated, the leucovorin must be increased (see below).

3. Dose and schedule of leucovorin administration:

(a) Leucovorin rescue must start 2 h following completion of MTX infusion.

(b) Leucovorin is given at a dose of 12 mg/m^2 IV every 3 h during the first 24 h for a total of eight doses. The same dose (12 mg/m^2) is continued every 6 h IM for the next 48 h or a total of eight additional doses. The first IM dose is given 3 h after the first IV dose.

(c) If, at 36 h, the serum creatinine continues to rise 50% or more above baseline values, or if the serum MTX level is above 1×10^{-7M}, institute 'super' leucovorin rescue at 100 mg/m^2 IM every 3 h until the serum MTX levels fall below 1×10^{-7M}.

(d) If the serum, MTX level does not rise above 1×10^{-7M} and the serum creatinine rises less than 50% above baseline values, but other signs of toxicity are present, such as oral ulcers, skin rash, etc., a further 48 h of leucovorin at 12 mg/m^2, every 6 h IM or PO should be given.

4. Pre-treatment evaluation:

(a) A complete history and physical examination is mandatory.

(b) Laboratory studies must include a WBC count with a full differential, platelet count, SMA, uric acid, Ca, P, serum creatinine and creatinine clearance, urinalysis.

(c) Chest X-ray. Full chest tomography to exclude effusions.

(d) A renal ultrasound or IVP should be obtained to rule out obstructive uropathy and to establish the presence of two functioning kidneys, if there is any doubt.

GENERAL GUIDELINE FOR THE ADMINISTRATION OF HIGH-DOSE MTX WITH LEUCOVORIN RESCUE (SUMMARY)

Hour:

−12:	Start intake of fluids, PO or IV. Start sodium bicarbonate, 3 g IV every 3 h for 60 h. Start measurements of urinary pH. Continue measurements on every voided sample. pH must be maintained at 7 or higher.
0:	If diuresis is adequate and urinary pH is 7 or higher, give MTX as a 6 h continuous IV infusion. Maintain IV fluids to assure total fluid intake of at least 3 litres in 24 h.
+8:	Start leucovorin rescue: 12 mg/m^2 every 3 h IV for 8 doses at 8,11,14,17,20,23,26,29 h).
+24:	Obtain serum creatinine and serum MTX levels.
+32:	Continue leucovorin rescue: 12 mg/m^2 every 6 h IM for 8 doses (at 32,38,44,50,56,62,74 h).
+36:	Obtain serum creatinine and serum MTX levels, if indicated. Modify leucovorin dose accordingly.
+48:	Obtain serum creatinine and serum MTX levels. If creatinine is normal, and serum MTX at non-toxic levels, IV fluids and bicarbonate may be discontinued.
+72:	Serum MTX levels.

IT administration of MTX: 0·15 – 0·25 mg/kg or 10 mg/m^2 (maximum 15 mg), may be given every 2–5 days until symptons of meningeal leukemia have cleared or signs of systemic toxicity occur.

Toxicity: ***Acute:*** Stomatitis, mild nausea.

Late: Stomatitis, common indicator for interruption of therapy. Diarrhoea; hemorrhagic enteritis with possible perforation; hepatic dysfunction, usually reversible but may lead to cirrhosis; occasional alopecia.

Central nervous system abnormalities with dizziness, blurred vision and even paresis and ataxia (following IT MTX). Myelosuppression is the dose-limiting toxicity, with leukopenia, anemia, and thrombocytopenia; leucovorin is the antedote for these phenomena and can be used to prevent them.

Renal complications are usually seen at the higher doses of MTX. Renal tubular necrosis with significant elevations in serum creatinine and blood urea nitrogen elevations occur if MTX is used in patients with prior renal impairment (see instructions forthe use of high-dose MTX and leucovorin rescue). Accordingly the renal status must be determined prior to MTX administration and followed carefully during treatment.

Alopecia and dermatitis are uncommon. Interstitial pneumonitis is uncommon but does occur.

METHYLHYDRAZINE

Synonyms: Procarbazine, [Matulane, Natulan]

Mechanism of Action: Monoamine oxidase inhibitor of DNA, RNA, and protein synthesis which is cell cycle phase non-specific. Auto-oxidation of the compound forms H_2O_2 and generates hydroxy radicals, leading to effects similar to ionizing radiation. The drug initially concentrates in the liver and kidney and is demethylated by hepatic microsomes and mostly excreted in the urine.

Administration: PO

Dosage: 1–2 mg/kg or 100 mg/m^2 per day. Patients who have received prior irradition or have a compromised bone-marrow should receive lower doses (1–2 mg/kg on alternate days). In the MOPP regimen it is given at 50 mg/day on day 1 and then escalated to 100 mg/m^2 on days 2–14.

Toxicity: ***Acute:*** stomatitis, diarrhoea and occasional dysphagia. Skin hypersensitivity reactions with eventual hyperpigmentation; facial flushing after alcohol ingestion, photophobia and photosensitivity may also occur. Jaundice is rare, while nausea and vomiting are dose-dependent. A flu-like syndrome, with myalgia, and arthralgia can develop.

Late: Central nervous system signs such as confusion, headache, depression, insomnia, paresthesiae and lethargy can occur. Myelosuppression with leukopenia and thrombocytopenia being most frequent, occurring between the second and fourth weeks after therapy.

MITHRAMYCIN

Synonym: [Mithracin]

Mechanism of Action: Antitumor antibiotic which is cell cycle phase non-specific, and its main activity is in the S-phase. The compound forms complexes with DNA, most specifically with guanine, particularly in the presence of divalent cations such as magnesium. DNA-dependent RNA synthesis is also inhibited. The drug appears to block resorption of calcium from bone with a direct effect on osteoclasts, thereby reducing plasma calcium levels. It is excreted in the urine and also crosses the blood-brain barrier.

Administration: IV

Dosage: 0·025–0·050 mg/kg may be given daily. If given on alternate days there is less hematopoetic toxicity.

It has also been used together with hydroxyurea without much success in the treatment of myeloid blast crisis of CGL. The drug is diluted in 0·25 or 0·5 litres 5% glucose in water, and given over 2–4 h. In this regimen it is given IV (25 μg/kg) every other day for 3 weeks together with 4 g hydroxyurea/day, provided the counts permitted this dosage.

Toxicity: ***Local:*** Irritating to the veins and surrounding tissue and extravastion should be avoided.

Acute: Nausea, vomiting, and anorexia are often severe and a metallic taste may be felt in the mouth, which can persist for 24–48 h. Hypocalcemia may be observed within 48 h of treatment and appropriate measures should be taken to prevent cardiotoxicity. Fever and facial flushing may also occur.

Late: Skin changes, facial erythema, edema, increased pigmentation and non-specific rashes occur.

Reversible hepatoxicity, with alterations of liver function tests are seen and decreased production of clotting factors and increased prothrombin times have been recorded.

Myelosuppression, and particularly thrombocytopenia may be of rapid onset, while leukopenia is rarer.

Hemorrhagic diathesis. The most serious toxicity may be uncontrolled spontaneous bleeding in the prescence of a normal platelet count and prothrombin time, particularly after higher cumulative doses have been used.

Abnormal renal function tests with renal failure and urologic irritability with lethargy may also occur.

MITOGUAZONE

Synonyms: Methyl GAG (methyl-glyoxal-bis-guanyl-hydrazone; MGBG)

Mechanism of Action: Interferes with the enzymes synthesizing physiologically active polyamines, in particular spermidine, which are involved in the initiation of DNA synthesis through stabilizing the DNA-polymerase–helix complex. The drug may cause spermidine depletion and putrescine accumulation which act to halt DNA synthesis and to block the activation (methylation) of transfer RNA. The drug is recovered in the urine after a prolonged time suggesting that there is an extravascular distribution.

Administration: IV

Dosage: 500 mg/m^2 given over 30–40 min once weekly. The dose can be escalated by 100 mg/m^2/week. A lower dose of 260 mg/m^2 week may also be used.

Local: Extravasation causes a severe local reaction with pain, inflammation, edema and ulceration.

Acute: Orthostatic hypotension occurs if the drug is given too quickly. A local burning sensation over the face and the entire body may develop with weakness and dizziness.

Late: Severe mucositis anorexia, weight loss, nausea, vomiting and diarrhea. Hypoglycemic reactions may also occur. Myelosuppression, occurs with leukopenia and thrombocytopenia being most frequent.

Neuropathy, myopathy and paralytic ileus are rare.

MITOXANTRONE

Synonym: [Novantrone] (Mitoxantrone HCl)

Mechanism of Action: Anthraquinone compound which belongs to the anthracenedione class, and is cell cycle non-specific. This compound, which lacks an amino-sugar moiety at the C9 position in the molecule, making it different to rubidazone or doxorubicin, is a DNA-reactive agent, excreted via the renal and hepatobiliary systems. The hepatobiliary elimination seems to be of greater significance. It intercalates into DNA and causes inter- and intra-strand cross-linking. It is believed to be associated with the inhibition of nucleic acid synthesis.

Administration: IV

Dosage: 10–14 mg/m^2 on days 1–3, in combination with other drugs for the induction of acute leukemia every 3–4 weeks. It can be used for 5 days as a single agent at 12 mg/m^2/day.

8 mg/m^2, a lower dose may be used in combination with other drugs, such as cyclophosphamide, etoposide and prednisone cyclically for the treatment of lymphoma. Others have used it at as much as 16 mg/m^2 IV for 5 days for relapsed leukemia and at 14 mg/m^2 IV as a single agent, every 3 weeks, for relapsed non-Hodgkin's lymphoma. Most recently the dosage has been escalated to much higher doses twice a day without undue toxicity.

Toxicity: ***Local:*** It has non-vesicant properties, which minimizes the likelihood of severe local recreations if extravasation should occur. Rare reports of tissue necrosis following extravasation have been recorded.

Immediate: Some nausea and vomiting.

Acute: Nausea, vomiting and anorexia occur in about 30% of patients and there is a green–blue discoloration of the urine.

Late: Mild alopecia occurs in about half the patients and phlebitis with blue discoloration of the veins occurs.

Bone-marrow suppression develops — mostly leukopenia and thrombocytopenia while anemia is less frequent.

Dose-limiting cardiotoxicity is rarely seen but may include ECG changes, arrhythmias, tachycardia and chest pain. Decreases in left ventricular ejection fraction have been recorded, but are rare. Congestive cardiac failure has been reported.

RUBIDAZONE

Synonym: Benzoyl hydrazone

Mechanism of Action: An anthracycline antibiotic which is semisynthetic. It is a class 3 cell cycle non-specific agent and is cumulative like other anthracyclines (see doxo- and daunorubicin). Most of the drug is excreted via the bile.

Administration: IV

Dosage: 8–16 mg/kg is the average dose. The cumulative dose is 3500 mg/m^2 if it is used alone, but the drug should be stopped at 1700 mg/m^2 in patients who have received previous anthracyclines. Cardiac monitoring must be used during the course of therapy and the ejection fraction should be assessed by echocardiogram or MUGA-scan.

Toxicity: ***Immediate:*** Allergic reactions, rash, anaphylaxis and fever with or without hypotension may occur.

Acute: Nausea, vomiting, and diarrhea are seen. Red urine (not hematuria) is evident.

Late: Mucositis is moderate, while alopecia is severe. Reactivation of radiation and previous skin problems, may develop during therapy. Myelosuppression occurs and is maximal after 2 weeks. Anthracycline cardiotoxicity is seen (See above dosage and data on other anthracyclines).

STREPTOZOTOCIN

Synonym: [Zanosar]

Mechanism of Action: Cell cycle phase non-specific but it appears to affect the S-phase mostly. The drug inhibits DNA synthesis directly, affecting pyrimidine nucleotides via potent inhibition. The drug inhibits enzymes involved in gluconeogenesis and is rapidly cleared from the plasma; it also crosses the blood–brain barrier. It is excreted in the urine.

Administration: IV

Dosage: 500 mg/m^2 IV for 1–5 days every 3–4 weeks, or 1 g/m^2 IV/week once every 4 weeks. The drug is contraindicated in renal disease or if renal toxicity occurs after previous administration of the drug. The creatinine clearance and albuminuria should be monitored.

Toxicity: *Local:* Local pain may occur at the site of injection, particularly if the infusion rate is too fast.

Acute: Nausea and vomiting may be very severe within an hour or two of administration of the drug.

Late: Nausea and vomiting may continue. Reversible hepatoxicity is usually mild with mild abnormalities in the liver function tests. Diarrhea is rare, as is hypoglycemia. Myelosuppression with anemia and leukopenia are more frequent than thrombocytopenia. Renal toxicity occurs with glycosuria and amino-aciduria, renal tubuclar acidosis and azotemia.

TENIPOSIDE

Synonyms: Epidophyllotoxin, VM-26, [Vumon]

Mechanism of Action: A plant alkaloid, which is a cell cycle phase-specific agent causing mitotic inhibition. It is a mitotic spindle poison in the M-phase and perhaps also active in late G_2-/M- interphase. Most of the compound is excreted via the biliary system while renal excretion is low.

Administration: IV

Dosage: 100–300 mg/m^2/week, sometimes in divided doses, infused over 30–60 min. 60 mg/m^2 IV for 4 day cycles has been used during consolidation therapy of ALL in the newer protocols.

Toxicity: *Local:* May be vesicant, and extravasation should be avoided.

Acute: Orthostatic hypotension occurs if the infusion is given too quickly. Moderate anorexia and nausea also occur.

Late: Nausea, vomiting and alopecia. Myelosuppression which is dose-limiting may develop with leucopenia, anemia and thrombocytopenia.

6-THIOGUANINE (6-TG)

Synonyms: 6-TG, 2-amino-6-mercaptopurine, [Lanvis]

Mechanism of Action: Antimetabolite, cell cycle S-phase-specific. This compound is an analog which specifically inhibits nucleic acid synthesis, after its conversion to a nucleotide, which is incorporated into DNA and to a lesser extent RNA. It substitutes for guanine, producing functionally altered polynucleotides thereby inhibiting the S-phase of the cell cycle. The compound is partially but rapidly absorbed from the gastrointestinal tract and is mostly excreted in the urine, within 24 h.

Administration: Mostly PO but can be used IV

Dosage: 2·0–2·5 mg/kg/day or twice daily together with Ara-C usually.

Toxicity: ***Immediate:*** None

Acute: Gastric intolerance with nausea and vomiting, diarrhea is rare.

Late: Nausea and vomiting are uncommon; stomatitis is rare. Occasional hepatic dysfunction occurs which is usually reversible with rare jaundice; Myelosuppression with leukopenia, thrombocytopenia and anemia with megaloblastosis.

THIOTEPA

Compound: Triethylene thiophosphopramide, Triethylene

Mechanism of Action: A trifunctional alkylating agent which is cell cycle non-specific, with an action very similar to that of mechorethamine. However it is not a vesicant. The drug is cleared from the plasma within a few minutes and most of it is excreted in the urine.

Administration: IV, IM (deep) and IC

Dosage: The usual systemic dose is 0·6–0·8 mg/kg given as a single or divided doses on successive days. Reduce the dosage when there is myelosuppression or if chemoradiotherapy has been given recently. 0·8 mg/kg of thiotepa is approximately equivalent to 0·4 mg/kg of mechlorethamine and 15–18 mg/m^2 has been used to substitue for mechlorethamine on days 1 and 8 of the MOPP regimen. Very high doses are now being used as part of a cytoreductive regimen before ABM transplantation.

IC administration is generally given at the same dose as above.

Toxicity: ***Local:*** Minimal toxicity, and it can be given by deep IM injection in patients with inaccessible veins.

Acute: Minimal nausea and vomiting with rare allergic reactions.

Late: Nausea, vomiting and anorexia may continue. Myelosuppression occurs with maximal leukopenia 10–14 days after injection. This may also occur after IC administration.

VINBLASTINE

Synonyms: [Velbe, Velban]

Mechanism of Action: It is a sulfate salt of the plant alkaloid derived from *Vinca rosea,* which interrupts mitotic spindle formation with specific action in the S-phase. It is a M-phase-specific drug, causing reversible mitotic arrest after binding to a cytoplasmic precursor of the spindle, during the S-phase. It also inhibits RNA synthesis via an effect on the DNA-dependent RNA polymerase system. The drug also causes rearrangement of the binding sites of microtubular units in the mitotic spindle with polymerization of the tubule structure.

The drug is rapidly cleared from the plasma within minutes and is primarily excreted in the bile. Some enterohepatic circulation occurs with excretion in the stool and urine.

Administration: IV

Dosage: 0·1–0·15 mg/kg weekly or biweekly or 6 mg/m^2. It can also be given at a higher dosage of 0·3–0·4 mg/kg IV every 3 weeks. Dose should be decreased in liver disease.

Toxicity: ***Local:*** Prolonged inflammatory reaction can occur with necrosis occuring on extravasation.

Acute: Nausea and vomiting occurs with occasional malaise, headache and paresthesiae. Jaw pain and occasional pain within the tumor area may develop, lasting from 20 min to 3 h.

Late: Myelosuppression and particularly leukopenia occurs within 5–10 days of administration. Thrombocytopenia is uncommon and anemia is rare. Occasional mild peripheral neuropathy, muscle weakness, areflexia, paralytic ileus and constipation occur but this is not as severe as with vincristine. Alopecia, mucositis and mental depression are rarely encountered.

VINCRISTINE

Synonym: [Oncovin]

Mechanism of Action: It is the sulfate salt of the dimeric vindoline catharanthine-like alkaloid derived from the plant *Vinca rosea*. It is cell cycle-specific and, like colchicine, blocks motisis with metaphase arrest. This specific M-phase inhibition is due to crystallization of the microtubular and spindle proteins. The drug has a rapid biphasic plasma clearance, is incompletely metabolized by the liver and excreted in the bile. There is an enteroheptic circulation with most of the drug excreted in the faeces and some in the urine.

Administration: IV

Dosage: 0·01–0·05 mg/kg or 1·0–1·4 mg/m^2 IV weekly in adults (no more than 2 mg per dose is *usually* given).

At the lower dose schedules, it may be possible to

give five or more weekly injections before neurotoxicity is reached. The dosage for children may be somewhat higher at 2 mg/m^2 weekly, without increased toxicity.

In recent years it has been given by continuous infusion, 1·0 mg/m^2 on days 1 and 2 or 0·4 mg/m^2 on days 1–4, particularly in the VAD regimen in myeloma.

Toxicity: ***Local:*** Severe local irritation occurs if it is injected SC.

Acute: Constipation and abdominal pain may develop which usually responds well to laxatives or enemas; if this is very severe it can be dose-limiting.

Late: Myelosuppression is very unusual and leukopenia is very rare.

Neurological findings including sensory neuropathy, sensory impairment and paresthesias occur (but these are not dose-limiting). However, severe paresthesiae, jaw pain, loss of deep tendon reflexes, ataxia, footdrop, altered gait and muscle wasting and paralytic ileus do occur and are dose limiting. Cranial nerve palsies are rare but can occur.

Alopecia occurs and inappropriate ADH secretion may develop rarely.

VINDESINE

Synonym: [Eldisine]

Mechanism of Action: Synthetic derivative of vinblastine, which is a phase-specific M-phase agent, excreted in the bile.

Administration: IV

Dosage: 2–4 mg/m^2 IV, weekly

Toxicity: ***Local:*** It is a vesicant, and locally irritating if injected SC; avoid extravasation.

Immediate: A cold sensation may develop in the vein on injection.

Acute: Some nausea and vomiting occurs which is transient, jaw pain may occur.

Late: Constipation and abdominal pain; mild to total alopecia, does occur.

Neurological toxicity, is similar to that for vincristine but is less severe and less common; Myelosuppression, particularly leukopenia with recovery after about a week does occur and can be dose-limiting. Thrombocytopenia is uncommon.

APPENDIX TO PART 1

The following tables may be useful to the treating physician giving chemotherapy.

Table 1. Recommended dose reduction in presence of myelosuppression on the day of drug administration

*Grade of toxicity**	*WBC*	*Platelets*	*Percentage of initial dose*
0	$>4\times10^9$/l	$>120\times10^9$/l	100 % all drugs
1	$2{\cdot}5$–$3{\cdot}99\times10^9$/l	80–119×10^9/l	100% of drugs not causing severe myelosuppression e.g. Bleomycin, Vincristine. 50% of all other drugs
2	$<2{\cdot}5\times10^9$/l	$<80\times10^9$/l	100 % of drugs not causing severe myelosuppression. All other drugs withheld until at least grade 1 toxicity is reached.

*See grade of toxicity scheme in Table 2

Reference

Hellmann, K. and Carter, S.K. (1987). *Fundamentals of Cancer Chemotherapy*. Reproduced with the permission of McGraw-Hill, Inc.

Table 2. Common dose change criteria by degree of myelosuppression

A. Level of lowest count ($\times 10^3$) recorded in previous course

Absolute no. of granulocytes		*No. of platelets*	*Dose change in next course*
>1·5		>150	50 % increase
1–1·5	and	100–150	25 % increase
0·5–0·9	and/or	50–99	No change
0·25–0·49	and/or	25–49	25 % decrease
<0·25	and/or	<25	50 % decrease

B. Regardless of count

Morbidity, e.g., significant infection and/or hemorrhage	50 % decrease

Reference

Hellmann, K. and Carter, S.K. (1987). *Fundamentals of Cancer Chemotherapy*. Reproduced with the permission of McGraw-Hill, Inc.

Table 3. Examples of general dose modifications in case of organ dysfunction in adults, particularly renal or hepatic function*

Altered Renal Function

Creatinine clearance ml/min/1·73	*Creatinine (mg/dl)*	*BUN (mg/dl)*	*Drug dosage (%)*
>70	<1–5	<20	100
50–70	1·5–2	20–50	50–75
<50	>2	>50	25–50

Altered Hepatic Function

Serum bilirubin (mg/dl)	*Other LFT***	*AN*** (%)*	*Other drugs (%)*
<1·2	<2 × normal	100	100
1·2–3	2·5 × normal	50	75
>3	> normal	25	50

*If liver severely involved by disease, some suggest a 50% dosage reduction of cytotoxic agents.
**Liver function tests = LFT
***Anthracycline = AN

Only approximate guidelines can be suggested and it must be obvious that the treating physician should adjust dosages according to each individual patient and disease instance.

Reference

Beretta, G. (1983). *Cancer Chemotherapy Regimens.* Reproduced with the permission of Farmitalia Carlo Erba Spa.

Table 4

Performance status (Karnofsky index)*

Able to carry on normal activity; no special care is needed

100 Normal no complaints, no evidence of disease.
90 Able to carry on normal activity; minor signs or symptoms of disease.
80 Normal activity with effort; some signs or symptoms of disease.

Unable to work; able to live at home; cares for most personal needs; a varying amount of assistance is needed

70 Cares for self; unable to carry on normal activity or do active work.
60 Requires occasional assistance, but is able to care for most of his/her needs.
50 Requires considerable assistance, and frequent medical care.

Unable to care for self; requires equivalent of institutional or hospital care; disease may be progressing rapidly

40 Disabled; requires special care and assistance.
30 Severely disabled; hospitalization is indicated, although death not imminent.
20 Very sick; hospitalization necessary.
10 Moribund; fatal process
0 Dead

Performance status (ECOG/WHO)†

0 Fully active able to carry out all pre-disease activities without restriction and without the aid of analgesia.

1 Restricted in strenuous activity but ambulatory and able to carry out light work or pursue a sedentary occupation. Patients who are fully active but require analgesia.

2 Ambulatory and capable of all self care but unable to carry out any work. Up and about more than 50% of waking hours.

3 Capable of only limited self care, confined to bed or chair more than 50% of waking hours.

4 Completely disabled. Unable to carry out any self care and confined totally to bed or chair.

5 Dead

Summary
0 Normal activity
1 Symptoms but ambulatory
2 In bed <50% of time
3 In bed > 50% of time
4 100% bed-ridden
5 Dead

References
*Karnofsky, D.A. and Burchenal, J.H. (1949). The clinical evaluation of chemotherapeutic agents. In *Evaluation of Chemotherapeutic Agents,* pp. 191–205. Edited by McLeod. New York: Columbia University Press.
†Miller, A.B., Hoogstaten, B., Staquet, M. and Winkler, A. (1981). Reporting results of cancer treatment. *Cancer* **47**, 207.

Table 5. Nomogram for determining body surface area of children and adults

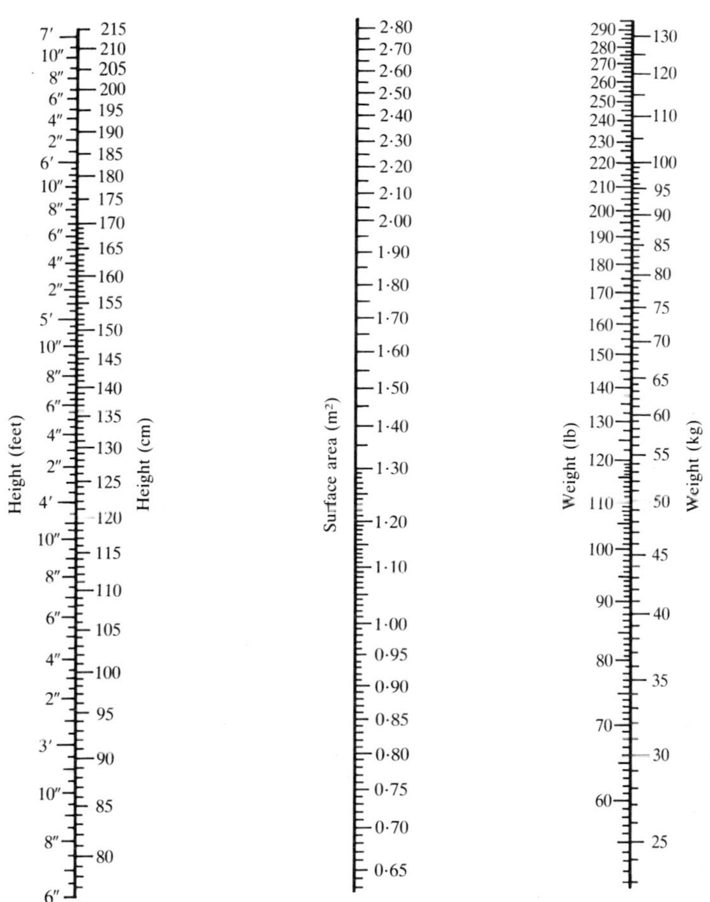

Body areas of both children and adults are indicated by intersection on the central scale of straight lines connecting weight and height values on the respective scales.

Reference

Boothby, W.M. and Sandiford, R.B. Reprinted by permission of The New England Journal of Medicine, **185:** 337 (1921).

Table 6. Definition of objective response in solid tumors

MEASURABLE DISEASE

Complete response
Disappearance of all known disease, determined by two observations not less than 4 weeks apart.

Partial response
50% or more decrease in total tumor load of the lesions that have been measured to determine the effect of therapy by two observations not less than 4 weeks apart. Measurement may be

(a) **bidimensional**
- single lesion: $\geq$ 50% decrease in tumor area (multiplication of longest diameter by the greatest perpendicular diameter);
- multiple lesions: a 50% decrease in the sum of the products of the perpendicular diameters of the multiple lesions.

(b) **unidimensional:** $\geq$ 50% decrease in linear tumor measurement.
In addition there can be no appearance of new lesions or progression of any lesion.

No change
A 50% decrease in total tumor size cannot be established nor has a 25% increase in the size of one or more measurable lesions been demonstrated.

Progressive disease
25% or more increase in the size of one or more measurable lesions or the appearance of new lesions.

NON-MEASURABLE DISEASE

Complete response
Complete disappearance of all known disease for at least 4 weeks.

Partial response
Estimated decrease in tumor size of $\geq$ 50% for at least 4 weeks.

No change
No significant change for at least 4 weeks. This includes stable disease, estimated decrease of $<$ 50%, and lesion with estimated increase of $<$ 25%.

Progressive disease
Appearance of any new lesions not previously identified or estimated increase of $\geq$ 25% in existent lesions.

Table 6. (continued)

BONE INVOLVEMENT

A separate set of response criteria are necessary for bone metastases.

Complete response
Complete disappearance of all lesions on x-ray or scan for at least 4 weeks.

Partial response
Partial decrease in size of lytic lesions, recalcification of lytic lesions, or decreased density of blastic lesions for at least 4 weeks.

No change
Because of the slow response of bone lesions, the designation of NC should not be applied until at least 8 weeks have passed from start of therapy.

Progressive disease
Increase in size of existent lesions or appearance of new lesions.

Occurrence of bone compression or fracture and its healing should not be used as the sole indicator for evaluation of therapy.

Reference

Miller, A.B., Hoogstaten, B., Staquet, M. and Winkler, A. (1981). Reporting results of cancer treatment. *Cancer* **47,** 207.

Table 7. Recommendation for grading of acute and subacute toxicity

	Grade 0	Grade 1	Grade 2	Grade 3	Grade 4
Hematologic (Adults)					
Hemoglobin (g/100 ml)	≥11·0	9·5–10·9	8·0–9·4	6·5–7·9	<6·5
Leukocytes $1000/mm^3$	≥4·0	3·0–3·9	2·0–2·9	1·0–1·9	<1·0
Granulocytes $1000/mm^3$	≥2·0	1·5–1·9	1·0–1·4	0·5–0·9	<0·5
Platelets $1000/mm^3$	≥100	75–99	50–74	25–49	<25
Hemorrhage	None	Petechiae	Mild blood loss	Gross blood loss	Debilitating blood loss
Gastrointestinal					
Bilirubin	≤1·25 × N*	1·26–2·5 × N	2·6–5 × N	5·1–10 × N	>10 × N
SGOT/SGPT	≤1·25 × N	1·26–2·5 × N	2·6–5 × N	5·1–10 × N	>10 × N
Alkaline phosphatase	≤1·25 × N	1·26–2·5 × N	2·6–5 × N	5·1–10 × N	>10 × N
Oral	None	Soreness/erythema	Erythema, ulcers, can eat solids	Ulcers, requires liquid diet only	Alimentation not possible
Nausea/vomiting	None	Nausea	Transient vomiting	Vomiting requiring therapy	Intractable vomiting
Diarrhoea	None	Transient <2 days	Tolerable but >2 days	Intolerable requiring therapy	Hemorrhagic dehydration

Table 7. (Continued)

Renal, bladder					
BUN or blood urea	≤ 1·25 × N	1·26–2·5 × N	2·6–5 × N	5–10 × N	> 10 × N
Creatinine	≤ 1·25 × N	1·26–2·5 × N	2·6–5 × N	5–10 × N	> 10 × N
Proteinuria	None	1 +, < 0·3 g/100 ml	2–3+, 0·3–1·0 g/100 ml	4+, > 1·0 g/100 ml	Nephrotic syndrome
Hematuria	None	Microscopic	Gross	Gross + clots	Obstructive uropathy
Pulmonary	None	Mild symptoms	Exertional dyspnea	Dyspnea at rest	Complete bed rest required
Fever (drug-induced)	None	Fever < 38°C	Fever 38°C–40°C	Fever > 40°C	Fever with hypotension
Allergic	None	Edema	Bronchospasm, no parental therapy needed	Bronchospasm, parental therapy required	Anaphylaxis
Cutaneous	None	Erythema	Dry desquamation, vesiculation, pruritus	Moist desquamation, ulceration	Exfoliative dermatitis, necrosis requiring surgical intervention
Hair	None	Minimal hair loss alopecia	Moderate, patchy alopecia	Complete alopecia but reversible	Non-reversible alopecia
Infection (specify size)	None	Minor infection	Moderate infection	Major infection	Major infection with hypotension

Table 7. (Continued)

	Grade 0	Grade 1	Grade 2	Grade 3	Grade 4
Cardiac					
Rhythm	None	Sinus tachycardia > 110 at rest	Unifocal PVC atrial arrythmia	Multifocal PVC	Ventricular tachycardia
Function	None	Asymptomatic, but abnormal cardiac sign	Transient symptomatic dysfunction, no therapy required	Symptomatic dysfunction responsive to therapy	Symptomatic dysfunction nonresponsive to therapy
Pericarditis	None	Asymptomatic effusion	Symptomatic, no tap required	Tamponade, tap required	Tamponade, surgery required
Neurotoxicity					
State of consciousness	Alert	Transient lethargy	Somnolence < 50% of waking hours	Somnolent > 50% of waking hours	Coma
Peripheral	None	Paresthesias and/or decreased tendon reflexes	Severe paresthesias and/or mild weakness	Intolerable paresthesias and/or marked motor loss	Paralysis
Constipation†	None	Mild	Moderate	Abdominal distention	Distention and vomiting
Pain‡	None	Mild	Moderate	Severe	Intractable

*N, upper limit of normal.

† Constipation does not include constipation resulting from narcotics.

‡ Pain – only treatment-related pain is considered, not disease-related pain. The use of narcotics may be helpful in grading pain, depending upon the tolerance level of the patient.

Reference

Miller, A.B., Hoogstaten, B., Staquet, M. and Winkler, A. (1981). Reporting results of cancer treatment. *Cancer* **47**, 210–211.

PART 2

CHEMOTHERAPY REGIMENS FOR HEMATOLOGICAL NEOPLASIAS

LYMPHOMA, LEUKEMIA AND MYELOMA

These are selected representative regimens which have been used successfully in the treatment of lymphomas, leukemias and myeloma. The absence of details of other regimens from this handbook does not imply that they are unsuccessful or not recommended for use. I have elected to include most of the conventional protocols and some of the alternative combinations and salvage regimens rather than list all the possible combinations used in every country, which obviously vary from center to center. On the other hand, the inclusion of the listed regimens does not imply that they have replaced others or that they are necessarily better than those excluded.

The details provided for these protocols are of necessity brief and are intended as aids rather than providing every detail. If there is any doubt about the dosage to be used or the days of administration I recommend the original references, most of which are listed.

Schedule modifications for dose attenuation of different drugs should be adhered to according to the outline given in the first part of the handbook or by the individual drug companies.

HODGKIN'S DISEASE

ABVD

Adriamycin	25 mg/m^2	IV	days 1 and 15
Bleomycin	10 mg/m^2	IV	days 1 and 15
Vinblastine	6 mg/m^2	IV	days 1 and 15
DTIC	375 mg/m^2	IV	days 1 and 15
	or		
	150 mg/m^2	IV	

No treatment given on days 16–28.

References

Bonadonna, G. *et al.* (1975). *Cancer* **36,** 252–259.

Sontoro, A. and Bonadonna, G. (1979). *Cancer Chemotherapy and Pharmacology* **2,** 101–105.

Cancer Treatment Rev. **9,** 21–35, 1982.

ABV

The same combination as ABVD without DTIC.
No treatment from days 15–28.

Alternating MOPP and ABV(D)

Mechlorethamine	6 mg/m^2	IV	days 1 and 8
Vincristine	1·4 mg/m^2	IV	days 1 and 8
Procarbazine	100 mg/m^2	PO	days 1–7
Prednisone*	40 mg/m^2	PO	days 1–14
Adriamycin	25 mg/m^2	IV	days 29 and 43
Bleomycin	10 mg/m^2	IV	days 29 and 43
Vinblastine	6 mg/m^2	IV	days 29 and 43
(DTIC)	150 mg/m^2	IV	days 29 and 43

No treatment from days 15–29, and 43–56.

Cycle frequency
MOPP and ABV(D) given on alternate months for 12 months.
*Prednisone given on cycles 1, 4, 7 and 10.

References
Bonadonna, G. *et al.* (1984). *Proc. Am. Soc. Oncol.* **3,** 254.
Bonadonna, G. *et al.* (1986). *Ann. Int. Med.* **104,** 739.

'Hybrid' MOPP/ABV(D)

Mechlorethamine	6 mg/m^2	IV	day 1
Vincristine	1·4 mg/m^2	IV	day 1
Procarbazine	100 mg/m^2	PO	days 1–7
Prednisone	40 mg/m^2	PO	days 1–14
Adriamycin	35 mg/m^2	IV	day 8
Bleomycin	10 mg/m^2	IV	day 8
Vinblastine	6 mg/m^2	IV	day 8
(DTIC)	150 mg/m^2	IV	day 8

No treatment given from day 14–28.

References
Klimo, P. and Connors, J.M. (1983). *Proc. Am. Soc. Clin. Oncol.* **2,** 208, (1985).
Klimo, P. *et al.* (1985). *J. Clin. Oncol.* 3, 1174.

B-CAVe*

Bleomycin	2·5 u/m^2	IV	days 1, 28 and 35
CCNU	100 mg/m^2	PO	day 1
Adriamycin	60 mg/m^2	IV	day 1
Vinblastine	5 mg/m^2	IV	day 1

No treatment given on days 36–42.
*Can also be given without Bleomycin as **CAVe**; no treatment on days 9–28.

References

Porzig, K.J., Portlock, C.S. *et al.* (1978). *Cancer* **41,** 1670–1675.
Harker, W. *et al.* (1984). *Ann. Int. Med.* **101,** 440–446.

BCVPP

BCNU	100 mg/m^2	IV	day 1
Cyclophosphamide	600 mg/m^2	IV	day 1
Vinblastine	5 mg/m^2	IV	day 1
Procarbazine	100 mg/m^2	PO	days 1–10
Prednisone	60 mg/m^2	PO	days 1–10

No treatment given on days 11–42.

Reference

Durant, J.R. *et al.* (1978). *Cancer* **42,** 2101–2110.

B-DOPA

Bleomycin	4 mg/m^2	IV	days 2 and 5
DTIC	150 mg/m^2	IV	days 1–5
Vincristine	1·5 mg/m^2	IV	days 1 and 5
Prednisone	40 mg/m^2	PO	days 1–6
Adriamycin	60 mg/m^2	IV	day 1

No treatment given on days 7–21 or 28.

Reference

Lokich, J.J. *et al.* (1976). *Cancer* **38,** 667–671.

B-MOPP (see listed under MOPP)

BVDS

Bleomycin	5 mg/m^2	IV	days 1 and 15
Vinblastine	6 mg/m^2	IV	days 1 and 15
Doxorubicin	30 mg/m^2	IV	day 1
Streptozotocin	1500 mg/m^2	IV	days 1 and 15

No treatment given from days 16–28.

Reference

Vinciguerra, V., Coleman, M. *et al.* (1977). *JAMA* **237,** 33–35.

CAVe

As in B-CAVe on p. 84 but without Bleomycin.

CEP

CCNU	80 mg/m^2	PO	day 1
Etoposide	100 mg/m^2	PO	days 1–5
Prednimustine*	60 mg/m^2	PO	days 1–5

No treatment given on days 6–28.
*Prednimustine may be replaced by Prednisone 40 mg/m^2 and Chlorambucil 6 mg/m^2 PO given on days 1–5.

References

Santoro *et al.* (1986). *Sem. Oncol.* **13** (Suppl), 23–26.
Cervantes, F. *et al.* (1986). *Cancer Treat. Rep.* **70,** 665–667.

CEVD

CCNU	80 mg/m^2	PO	day 1
Etoposide	120 mg/m^2	PO	days 1–5 and
	or		days 22–26
	60 mg/m^2	IV	
Vindesine	3 mg/m^2	IV	days 1 and 22
Dexamethasone	3 mg/m^2	PO	days 1–8
	1·5 mg/m^2	PO	days 9–26

No treatment is given from days 27–42.

Reference
Pfreundschuch, N.G. *et al.* (1987). *Cancer Treat. Rep.* **71,** 1203–1207.

ChlVPP

Chlorambucil	6 mg/m^2 (not exceeding 10 mg/day)	PO	days 1–14
Vinblastine	6 mg/m^2	IV	days 1 and 8
Procarbazine	100 mg/m^2	PO	days 1–14
Prednisolone	40 mg/m^2 (25 mg/m^2 in children)	PO	days 1–14

Comments
No treatment on days 15–28.
Cycles are given until remission is obtained and then five further cycles are given.

References
McElwain, T.J. *et al.* (1981). *Brit. J. Cancer* **36,** 276–280.
Daly, R.J., McElwain, T.J. *et al.* (1982). *Brit. J. Cancer* **45,** 851–859.

CMMVEP

Cyclophosphamide	400 mg/m^2	IV	day 1
Mitoxantrone	8 mg/m^2	IV	day 1
MTX	30 mg/m^2	IV	day 8
Vincristine	2 mg	IV	day 8
Etoposide	100 mg/m^2	PO	days 14 and 15
Prednisolone	40 mg/m^2	PO	days 1–21

Given every 35 days with no therapy from day 22–35, as a weekly low-dose regimen, for 3–6 cycles; as used in Royal Marsden Hospital, London, UK.

C-MOPP (See listed under MOPP)

CVPP (C = CCNU)

CCNU	75 mg/m^2	PO	day 1
Vinblastine	4·5 mg/m^2	IV	days 1 and 8
Procarbazine	100 mg/m^2	PO	days 1–14
Prednisone*	40 mg/m^2	PO	days 1–14

No treatment given from days 15–28.
*Prednisone on cycles 1 and 4 only.

Reference

Cooper, M.R. *et al.* (1980). *Cancer* **46,** 654–662.

CVPP (C = cyclophosphamide)

Cyclophosphamide	300 mg/m^2	IV	days 1 and 8
Vinblastine	10 mg	IV	days 1, 8, 15
Procarbazine	100 mg/m^2	PO	days 1–14
Prednisone*	40 mg/m^2	PO	days 1–14

No treatment given from days 16–42.
*Prednisone on cycles 1 and 4 only.

Reference
Bloomfield, C.D. *et al.* (1976). *Cancer* **38,** 42–48.

CVPP (**C** = cyclophosphamide)

Cyclophosphamide	600 mg/m^2	day 1
Vinblastine	6 mg/m^2	day 1
Procarbazine	100 mg/m^2	days 1–14
Prednisone*	40 mg/m^2	days 1–14

No treatment given from days 15–28.
*Prednisone on cycles 1 and 4 only.

Reference
Morgenfeld, M. *et al.* (1979). *Cancer* 43, 1579–1586.

EBVP

Epirubicin	70 mg/m^2	IV	day 1
Bleomycin	10 mg/m^2	IV	day 1
Vinblastine	6 mg/m^2	IV	day 1
Prednisolone	40 mg/m^2	IV	day 1 then PO day 2–5

No treatment given from days 6–22.

Reference
Hoerni B. *et al. (1987) Proc. Am. Soc. Clin. Oncol.* **6**: A743.
Zittoun R. *et al. (1987) Bull. Cancer,* **74**: 151–157.

Alternating EBV/C – MOPP

Epirubicin	30 mg/m^2	IV	days 1+15
Bleomycin	10 mg/m^2	IM	days 1+15
Vinblastine	6 mg/m^2	IV	days 1+15

C-MOPP every 28 days (see page 101)
No treatment given from days 16–28.

Reference
Tedeschi L. *et al. 3rd International Conference on Malignant Lymphoma,* Lugano, June 10–13, 1987. Abstracts, p 133

HOPE – BLEO

Doxorubicin	40 mg/m^2	IV	day 1
Vincristine	1·4 mg/m^2	IV	days 1 and 8
Prednisolone	100 mg	PO	days 1–8
Etoposide	200 mg/m^2	PO	days 1–4 (5)
Bleomycin	10 mg/m^2	IV	days 1 and 8

No treatment given on days 9–21 or 28.

Reference
McElwain, T.J. *et al.* (1986). Proc. of Workshop on the role of epidophyllotoxins in cancer chemotherapy, *14th Int. Congress on Chemotherapy 1985,* 29–36.

IMEP

Ifosfamide*	1000 mg/m^2	IV	days 1–5
MTX	30 mg/m^2	IV	day 3
Etoposide	100 mg/m^2	IV	days 1–3
Prednisone	40 mg/m^2	PO	days 1–7

This regimen has been given as the third cycle sequentially after COPP (days 1–14) and ABV (day 15), starting on day 29. No treatment given from days 36–43.
**MESNA* should be given with ifosfamide.

Reference
Diehl, V., (1988). *BMET study for Hodgkin's lymphoma,* University Clinic, Köln, West Germany.

Mini – BEAM

Carmustine	60 mg/m^2	IV	day 1
Etoposide	75 mg/m^2	IV	days 2–5
Cytosine arabidoside	100 mg/m^2	IV	days 2–5
Melphalan	30 mg/m^2	IV	day 6

No treatment given from days 7–28.

Reference
As used at University College Hospital, London, UK by A.H. Goldstone *et al.* and as in Stewart A.K. *et al. Leukemia & Lymphoma:* **5**: (2 & 3), 1991.

MOPP

Mechlorethamine	6 mg/m^2		days 1 and 8
Vincristine	1·4 mg/m^2	IV	days 1 and 8
Procarbazine	100 mg/m^2	PO	days 1–14
Prednisone*	40 mg/m^2	PO	days 1–14

No treatment given on days 15–28.
*Prednisone is only given on cycles 1–4.

References
De Vita, V.T. *et al* (1970). *Ann. Int. Med.* **73,** 881–895.
Longo, D.L. *et al.* (1986). *J. Clin. Oncol.* **4,** 1295.

B-MOPP

Same regimen as in MOPP but low dose. Bleomycin is added 2 mg/m^2 IV on days 1 and 8.
Procarbazine may be shortened to days 1–10.
No treatment from days 15–28.

Reference
Grozea, P.N. *et al.* (1985). *Malignant Lymphomas and Hodgkin's Disease: Experimental and Therapeutic Advances,* p. 346. Boston: Martinus Nijhoff.

C-(M)OPP

As in MOPP but no or alternating mechlorethamine.
Cyclophosphamide given IV 650 mg/m^2 on days 1 and 8 (instead of mechlorethamine). (See page 101)
No treatment from days 15–28.

Reference
De Vita V.T. (1975) *Lancet* **1,** 248–250.

T-MOPP

Same regimen as MOPP but *instead* of mechlorethamine, *Thiotepa* is given 15 mg/m^2 IV on days 1 and 8. No treatment given on days 15–28.

MVPP

As in MOPP but with the following changes:
Vinblastine (Velban) 6 mg/m^2 IV on days 1 and 8, instead of Vincristine.
No treatment is given from days 15–42.

References
McElwain, T.J. (1974). *et al. National Cancer Inst. Monograph* **36,** 395–402.
Sutcliffe, S.B. *et al.* (1978) *Brit. Med. J.* **1,** 679–683.

NOVP

Novantrone	8 mg/m^2	IV	day 1
Oncovin	2 mg	IV	day 8
Vinblastine	6 mg/m^2	IV	day 1
Prednisone	100 mg/m^2	PO	days 1–5

No treatment from day 8–21.

Reference
Hagemeister, F. *et al. Fourth International Conference on Malignant Lymphoma,* June 6–9, 1990, p. 24. Lugano, Switzerland.

PAVe

Procarbazine	100 mg/m^2	PO	days 1–14
Alkeran	7·5 mg/m^2	PO	days 1 & 2; 8 & 9
Vinblastine	6 mg/m^2	IV	days 1 and 8

No treatment given from days 15–28.

Reference

Wolin, E.M. and Rosenberg, S.A. (1979). In *Adjuvant Therapy of Cancer II, pp. 119–127.* Edited by S.E. Salmon and S.E. Jones. New York: Grune and Stratton.

SCAB

Streptozotocin	500 mg/m^2	IV	days 1–5
CCNU	100 mg/m^2	PO	day 1
Adriamycin	45 mg/m^2	IV	day 1
Bleomycin	15 mg/m	IM	days 1–8

No treatment given between days 9–28.

Reference

Diggs, C.H., Wiernik, P.H. *et al.* (1981). *Cancer* **47,** 224–228.

T-MOPP (See listed under MOPP)

VEEP

Vincristine	1·4 mg/m^2	IV	days 1 and 8
Epirubicin	50 mg/m^2	IV	day 1
Etoposide	200 mg/m^2 or	IV	days 1–4
	(100 mg/m^2)	PO	days 1–8
Prednisone	40 mg/m^2	PO	days 1–8

No treatment given on days 9–21.

Reference

Cunningham D., Mansi J.L., *Pharmorubicin Update 90,* Symposium Proceedings, July 1990, pp. 44–45.

NON-HODGKIN'S LYMPHOMA

ACOMLA

As *COMLA* but some protocols have added ***Adriamycin*** 40 mg/m^2 IV on day 1 and dropped the cyclophosphamide to 1·0 g/m^2 IV.

Reference
Todd, M., Cadman, E. *et al.* (1984). *J. Clin. Oncol.* **2,** 986–993.

BACOP

Bleomycin	5 mg/m^2	IV	days 15 and 22
Adriamycin	25 mg/m^2	IV	days 1 and 8
Cyclophosphamide	650 mg/m^2	IV	days 1 and 8
Oncovin	1·4 mg/m^2	IV	days 1 and 8
Prednisone	60 mg/m^2	PO	days 15–28

Cycles given every 28 days for at least 6 cycles.

Reference
Schein *et al.* (1975). *Ann. Int. Med.* **85,** 417–422.

Other **BACOP** *regimens* have also been used e.g.

Bleomycin	5 mg/m^2	IV	days 1 and 5
Adriamycin	50 mg/m^2	IV	day 1
Cyclophosphamide	750 mg/m^2	IV	day 1
Vincristine	1·4 mg/m^2	IV	days 1 and 5
Prednisone	100 mg/m^2	PO	days 1–5.

No treatment given on days 6–21.
6–9 cycles given.

Reference
Skarin *et al.* (1977). *Blood* **49,** 759–770.

CEMP

Mitoxantrone	8 mg/m^2	IV	day 1
Etoposide	150 mg/m^2	IV	day 1
Cis-platinum	20 mg/m^2	IV	days 1–5
Prednisone	40 mg/m^2	PO	days 1–5

No treatment on days 6–21.

Reference
Chisesi, T. *et al.* *4th International Conference on Malignant Lymphoma, June 6–9 1990.* Lugano, Switzerland.

CEOP

Cyclophosphamide	750 mg/m^2	IV	day 1
Epirubicin*	60 mg/m^2	IV	day 1
Vincristine	1.5 g/m^2	IV	day 1
Prednisolone*	60 mg/m^2	PO	days 1–5

8 courses at 3 weekly intervals

Reference
Al-Ismail S.A.D., Whittaker J.A. and Gough. J. (1987). *Eur. J. Cancer Clin. Oncol.* **23**: 1379–1384

*In other protocols it is given as above but with epirubicin at 50 mg/m^2 on day 1 and 100 mg prednisolone PO on days 1–5.

Reference
Abate G. *et al.* (1987). *Tumori* **73**: 43–47

CEOP

Cyclophosphamide	600 mg/m^2	IV	days 1+8
Epirubicin	30 mg/m^2	IV	days 1+8
	(or 50 mg/m^2	IV	day 1)
Vincristine	1·4 mg/m^2	IV	days 1+8
Prednisolone	100 mg	PO	days 1–5

Repeat every 3–4 weeks

Reference

Sun Y. et al. 3rd International Conference on Malignant Lymphoma, Lugano, June 10–13, 1987. Abstracts, no. T144

Even higher doses of Epirubicin have been used: 50–70 mg/m^2 on day 1 in **CEOP(B)** and 90 mg/m^2 on day 1 in **High dose CEOP.**

References

De Lena M. *et al. Clin. Trials J.* **24** (suppl 1): 223–229, 1987
Lambertenghi-Deliliers G. *et al. 4th European Conference on Clinical Oncology and Cancer Nursing, Madrid, Nov 1–4, 1987,* Abstracts, p 26–27

CHOP

Cyclophosphamide	750 mg/m^2	IV	day 1
Adriamycin	50 mg/m^2	IV	day 1
Vincristine	1·4 mg/m^2	IV	day 1
Prednisone	25 mg, q.i.d.	PO	days 1–5

No treatment given between days 6–21.
At least 6 cycles given.

Reference

McKelvey, E.M. *et al.* (1975). *Proc. Am. Soc. Clin. Oncol.* **16,** 223.

CHOP-BLEO

Same as CHOP but with the addition of *Bleomycin** 10 mg/m^2 IV on days 1 and 5.
Vincristine is given again at same dose in CHOP on day 5. No treatment given from day 6–21.

**Bleomycin* is reduced to 4 mg/m^2 on days 1 and 5 for patients older than 60 years.

Reference
Rodriguez, V. et al. (1977). *Blood* **49,** 325–333.

CHOP-BLEO

Alternative dosages to those described above:

Cyclophosphamide	600 mg/m^2	IV	day 1
Adriamycin	40 mg/m^2	IV	day 1
Vincristine	2 mg/m^2	IV	day 1
Bleomycin	5 mg/m^2	IV	day 1
Prednisone	40 mg/m^2	PO	days 1–5

No treatment given on days 6–21.

Reference
Flippin, T. *et al.* (1983). *Cancer* **51,** 987–993.

C-MOPP (See COPP)

COMLA

Cyclophosphamide	1·5 g/m^2	IV	day 1
Vincristine	1·4 mg/m^2	IV	days 1, 8 and 15
MTX	120 mg/m^2	IV	days 22, 29, 36, 43, 50, 57, 64 and 71
Leucovorin	25 mg/m^2	PO	every 6 h × 6 starting 24 h after MTX
Ara-C	300 mg/m^2	IV	days as for MTX

No treatment given from day 72–86.
At least 3 cycles given.

Reference
Sweet, D.L., Golomb H.M., *et al.* (1980). *Ann. Int. Med.* **92,** 785–790.

COP

Cyclophosphamide*	800 mg/m^2	IV	day 1
Oncovin	2 mg	IV	day 1
Prednisone**	60 mg/m^2	PO	days 1–5

**Then 3 days of decreasing dosage of 40, 20, 10 mg/m^2, on days 6–8.
Treatment is not given from day 9–14; at least 6 cycles are given.
*(400 mg/m^2 if bone-marrow impaired).

Reference
Luce, J.K. *et al.* (1971). *Cancer* **26 (2),** 306–317.

COPBLAM

Cyclophosphamide*	400 mg/m^2	IV	day 1
Vincristine	1 mg/m^2	IV	day 1
Prednisone	40 mg/m^2	PO	days 1–10
Bleomycin	15 mg/m^2	IV	day 14
Adriamycin*	40 mg/m^2	IV	day 1
Procarbazine	100 mg/m^2	PO	days 1–10

No treatment between days 15–21.
At least 8 cycles are given.
*Includes escalation of cyclophosphamide by 100 mg/m^2 each cycle to a maximum of 700 mg/m^2 and Adriamycin by 10 mg each cycle to a maximum of 70 mg/m^2.
Consult reference for dose escalation.

Reference
Laurence, J., Coleman, M. *et al.* (1982). *Ann. Int. Med.* **97,** 190–195.

COPBLAM II

Essentially as above with continuous infusion of *bleomycin* 7·5 mg/m^2 over 24 h for 5 days, and vincristine 1 mg/m^2 continuous IV infusion over 24 h for 2 days.

Reference
Hollister, D., Silver, R.T. *et al.* (1982). *Cancer* **50,** 1690–1694.

COPBLAM III

Cyclophosphamide	350 mg/m^2	IV	days 1 and 22
Oncovin	1 mg/m^2	IV	continuous infusion over 24 h on days 1 and 2 and IV bolus on day 22
Prednisone	40 mg/m^2	PO	days 1–5; and on days 22–27
Bleomycin	7·5 mg/m^2	IV	push on day 1 (and then as a continuous infusion over 24 h from day 2), days 1–5
Adriamycin	35 mg/m^2	IV	days 1 and 22
Procarbazine	100 mg/m^2	PO	days 1–5 and 22–27

Treatment is not given on days 6–21 and from days 28–42.
Treatment given for 6 cycles. Each cycle is 42 days.

Doses of Adriamycin were escalated by 5 mg each cycle to a maximum of 50 mg/m^2 and cyclophosphamide by 50 mg each cycle to a maximum of 500 mg/m^2 dose.

Dose modifications – see original reference.

Reference
Boyd, D.B., Coleman, M. *et al.* (1988). *J. Clin. Oncol.* **6,** 425–433.

COPP (C-MOPP)

Cyclophosphamide	650 mg/m^2	IV	days 1 and 8
Oncovin	1·4 mg/m^2	IV	days 1 and 8
Procarbazine	100 mg/m^2	PO	days 1–10
Prednisone*	40 mg/m^2	PO	days 1–14

From day 14–28 no treatment given. 6–8 cycles given.
*Prednisone given only in cycles 1 and 4.

Reference
De Vita, V.T. *et al.* (1975). *Lancet* **1,** 248–250.

Cyclophosphamide may be used alternatively with mechlorethamine (6 mg/m^2) IV on days 1 and 8 in the same regimen as above, often termed C-MOPP.

CPOB

Cyclophosphamide	1000 mg/m^2	IV	day 1
Prednisone	100 mg/m^2	PO	days 1–5
Oncovin	1·2 mg/m^2	IV	day 15
Bleomycin	10 mg/m^2	IV	day 15

No treatment given on days 16–21.

Reference
Johnson, G.J. *et al.* (1983). *Cancer* **52,** 1133–1141.

CVP

Cyclophosphamide	400 mg/m^2	PO	days 1–5
Vincristine	1·4 mg/m^2	IV	day 1
Prednisone	100 mg/m^2	PO	days 1–5

No treatment given on days 6–21.
At least 6–8 cycles are given.

Reference

Bagley, C.M., De Vita, V.T. *et al.* (1972). *Ann. Int. Med.* **78,** 227–234.

DICE

Dexamethasone	10 mg IV 6h	days 1–4
Ifosamide	1·0 g/m^2 (with 1·75 g maximum) in 100 ml normal saline over 15 min.	days 1–4
Cisplatin	25 mg/m^2 in 250 ml normal saline over 1 h.	days 1–4
Etoposide	100 mg/m^2 in 500 ml normal saline over 1 h.	days 1–4
MESNA bolus	200 mg/m^2 in 50 ml normal saline over 5 min, 1 h prior to each ifosfamide.	days 1–4
MESNA infusion	300 mg/m^2 in 1 liter normal saline over 7 h × 3 bags daily.	days 1–4

NOTE: on day 4 MESNA runs for only 14 h after the last dose of ifosfamide.

Anti-emetics

Metoclopramide 20 mg 1 h pre-etoposide then every 2h × 3 post-chemotherapy.

Reference
Nichols, C.R. *et. al.* (1988) *Med. Ped. Oncol.* **16**: 12–16.
Haim, N. *et. al.* (1990) *Ann. Oncol.* **1(4)** (Abstract p 1–12).
Goss, P.E. *et. al.* (1991) *Ann. Oncol.* **2(1):** 43–46.

HOAP – BLEO

Adriamycin	40 mg/m^2	IV	day 1
Oncovin	1·4 mg/m^2	IV	day 1
Ara-C	14 mg/m^2	SC	q. 6 h (20 injections)
Prednisone	100 mg	PO	days 1–5
Bleomycin	15 units	IM	days 1–5

No treatment on days 6–21 or 28.

Reference
Cabanillas, F. *et al.* (1983). *Am. J. Med.* **74,** 382–388.

F-MACHOP

Vincristine	0·5 mg/m^2	IV	q. 12 h on day 1
Cyclophosphamide	800 mg/m^2	IV	after 24 h on day 2
5-Fluorouracil	15 mg/kg	IV	over 6 h on day 2 (at 36–42 h)
Ara-C	1·0 g/m^2	IV	over 6 h (at 42–48 h) on day 2
Adriamycin	60 mg/m^2	IV	12 h later (at 48 h) on day 3 (40 mg/m^2 IV is given during cycles 4–6)
MTX	500 mg/m^2	IV	over 6 h (during 60–66 h) on day 3 (300 mg/m^2 is given during cycles 4–6)
Leucovorin	20 mg/m^2	IV	after 24 hrs, IV, ev. 6h × 6
Prednisone	60 mg/m^2	PO	days 1–4

Prophylactic IT MTX 12 mg (total dose) and Ara-C 30 mg/m^2 is given on day 10. Cycles are given every 21–28 days.

Reference
Amadori, S. *et al.* (1985). *Sem. Oncol.* **12,** no. 2, Suppl. 2, 218–222.

MACOP – B

MTX*	400 mg/m^2	IV	during weeks 2, 6 and 10
Adriamycin	50 mg/m^2	IV	during weeks 1, 3, 5, 7, 9 and 11
Cyclophosphamide	350 mg/m^2	IV	during weeks 1, 3, 5, 7, 9 and 11
Oncovin	1·4 mg/m^2	IV	during weeks 2, 4, 6, 8, 10 and 12
Prednisone†	75 mg/m^2	PO	daily during weeks 1–12
Bleomycin	10 mg/m^2	IV	during weeks 4, 8 and 12

*MTX given as 100 mg/m^2 IV bolus, then 300 mg/m^2 IV over 4 h followed 24 h later by leucovorin 15 mg PO every 6 h for 6 doses.

†Tapered over the last 15 days.

Therapy is completed after 12 weeks.

Schedule is given weekly irrespective of severe thrombocytopenia. Repeated sepsis with neutropenia will result in schedule delay.

Reference
Klimo, P. and Connors, J.M. (1985). *Ann. Int. Med.* **102,** 596–602.

m-BACOD

MTX*	200 mg/m^2	IV	days 8 and 15 followed in 24 h by Leucovorin 10 mg/m^2 IV every 6 h × 6
Bleomycin	4 mg/m^2	IV	day 1
Adriamycin	45 mg/m^2	IV	day 1
Cyclophosphamide	600 mg/m^2	IV	day 1
Vincristine	1·0 mg/m^2	IV	day 1
Dexamethasone	6 mg/m^2	PO	days 1–5

No treatment given between day 15–21.
Ten cycles are usually given.

Reference
Skarin, A. (1983). *Proc. Am. Soc. Clin. Oncol.* **2,** 220.

M*-BACOD is given as above but with higher doses of MTX which are given only on day 14 at 3 g/m^2 IV.
Leucovorin is then given in a different schedule at 12 mg/m^2 IV 24 h after MTX, then every 3 and later 6 h for 72 h (see also pages 52–56).

Reference
Skarin, A.T., Cannellos G.P. *et al.* (1983). *J. Clin. Oncol.* **1,** 91–98.

MECOP-B

See **MACOP(B)** with epirubicin 75 mg/m^2 instead of Adriamycin.

Reference
Ibrahim E.M. *et al. Eur. J. Can. Clin. Oncol.* **23**: 391–401, 1988

PROMACE – CYTABOM

Etoposide	120 mg/m^2	IV	day 1
Adriamycin	25 mg/m^2	IV	day 1
Cyclophosphamide	650 mg/m^2	IV	day 1
MTX	120 mg/m^2	IV	day 8 (followed by Leucovorin PO for 2 days, given as in other schedules)
Prednisone	60 mg/m^2	PO	from days 1–14
Ara-C	300 mg/m^2	IV	day 8
Bleomycin	5 mg/m^2	IV	day 8
Vincristine	1·4 mg/m^2	IV	day 8

No treatment given from days 14–21 or 28.
6–8 cycles are given.

References

Fisher, R.I., De Vita, V.T. *et al.* (1984). *Proc. Am. Soc. Clin. Oncol.* **3,** 242.
Casciato, D.A. and Lowitz, B.B. (1989). *Manual of Clinical Oncology,* 2nd edn, p. 335. Boston, Mass.: Little Brown & Co.

PROMACE – MOPP

Etoposide	120 mg/m^2	IV	days 1 and 8, infused over a minimum of 1h
Cyclophosphamide	650 mg/m^2	IV	days 1 and 8
Adriamycin	25 mg/m^2	IV	days 1 and 8
MTX*	1·5 g/m^2	IV	over 12 h on day 14
with Leucovorin	50 mg/m^2	IV	every 6 h × 5 starting 24 h after MTX on day 15
Prednisone	60 mg/m^2	PO	days 1–14

No therapy given between days 15–28.

Comments
Initial therapy given for a number of cycles, depending on clinical response followed by a variable number of *MOPP cycles,* given as for regular MOPP (page 91). This is *flexitherapy*; MOPP may also be given *alternating* with PROMACE every 28 days.

At least 6 cycles are given. In some PROMACE, maintenance (intensification) is given every 56 days.

**MTX* at 500 mg/m^2 may also be used instead of 1·5 g/m^2.

Reference
Fisher, R.I., De Vita, V.T. *et al.* (1983). *Ann. Int. Med.* 98, 304–309.

'Hybrid' PROMACE – MOPP

Etoposide	120 mg/m^2	IV	day 1
Cyclophosphamide	650 mg/m^2	IV	day 1
Adriamycin	25 mg/m^2	IV	day 1
MTX	500 mg/m^2	IV	day 14
(Leucovorin given as in regular protocol)			
Prednisone	60 mg/m^2	PO	days 1–14
Mechlorethamine	6 mg/m^2	IV	day 8
Vincristine	1·4 mg/m^2	IV	day 8
Procarbazine	100 mg/m^2	PO	days 8–14

No treatment on days 16–28.
Mininum of 6 cycles.

VACOP – B

Etoposide (VP-16)	50 mg/m^2	IV	on day 1
	100 mg/m^2	PO	on days 2 & 3 during weeks 3, 7, 11
Adriamycin	50 mg/m^2	IV	weeks 1, 3, 5, 7, 9, 11
Cyclophosphamide	350 mg/m^2	IV	weeks 1, 5, 9
Oncovin	1·2 mg/m^2	IV	weeks 2, 4, 6, 8, 10, 12
Prednisone*	45 mg/m^2	PO	daily weeks 1 to 12
Bleomycin**	10 mg/m^2	IV	weeks 2, 4, 6, 8, 10, 12

Therapy is completed after 12 weeks.

*Prednisone given daily for the first week and then every second day for the next 11 weeks.

**Bleomycin given with 100 mg hydrocortisone IV.

Patients with bone marrow involvement will receive prophylactic *intrathecal* therapy (IT) with 12 mg methotrexate (IT) and cytosine arabinoside (IT) 30 mg/m^2 twice a week for 6 doses after the bone marrow involvement has resolved. After IT therapy 15 mg folinic acid should be given.

No dose modifications are used for thrombocytopenia.
If granulocyte count is 100–999/mm^3, 65% of cytotoxic drug dose is given; if granulocytes are $<$ 100/mm^3 postpone therapy for a week.

Reference

Connors, J.M., Hoskins, P., Klasa, R. *et al.* (1990). *Proc. ASCO.* **9**, 254 (abstract 983).

VEP

Vindesine	3 mg/m^2	IV	day 1 and 8
Etoposide	100 mg/m^2	IV	day 1
	200 mg/m^2	PO	days 2–3
Prednisone	25 mg/m^2	PO	days 1–7

No treatment from days 8–21.

Reference

Hancock, B.W. (1985). *Sem. Oncol.* **12,** 26–28.

SOME SALVAGE REGIMENS FOR LYMPHOMAS*

*Some of these regimens are used as salvage protocols for cytoreduction, before bone marrow transplantation.

CiEP

Cis-platinum	60 mg/m^2	IV	day 1
Etoposide	120 mg/m^2	PO	days 3–5
Prednisone	60 mg/m^2	PO	days 1–5

No treatment given from days 6–21.

Reference
Cavalli, F. (1985). *Sem. Oncol.* **12,** 33–36.

CPA-D

Cis-platinum	100 mg/m^2	IV	days 1 and 2
Ara-C	1 g/m^2		q. 12 h on days 1 and 2
Dexamethasone	40 mg/m^2	PO	days 1–4

No treatment on days 5–21 or 28.

References
Cabanillas, F. *et al.* (1988). *Blood* **71,** 117.
Cabanillas, F. (1989). *Sem. Oncol.* **16,** 78.

DHAP

Hydration with normal saline solution with *Mannitol* 50 g/l at 250 cm^2/h over 36 h.

After the first 6 h of hydration:

Cisplatin	100 mg/m^2	IV over	24 h on day 1
Ara-C	2 g/m^2	3 h infusion	q. 12 h on day 2
Dexamethasone	40 mg	PO/IV	days 1–4

Cycle given every 21–28 days.

Reference
Velasquez, W.S. *et al.* (1988). *Blood* **71,** 117–112.

DICE (As listed on page 102)

ESAP

Etoposide	60 mg/m^2	IV	days 1–4
Methylprednisolone	500 mg/m^2	IV	days 1–4
Ara-C (high-dose)	2 g/m^2	IV	day 4
Cis-platinum	100 mg/m^2	IV	continuous infusion days 1–4

No treatment from days 5–21.

Reference
Cabanillas, F., Rodriguez, M.A., *et al. Fourth International Conference on Malignant Lymphoma, June 6–9, 1990.* Lugano, Switzerland.

HAM

Ara-C* (high-dose)	3 g/m^2	IV	q. 12 h days 1–2
Mitoxantrone*	10 mg/m^2	IV	days 3–5

No treatment from days 6–14 or 28.

**Subsequent escalations* comprised 6–8 doses of HiDAC on days 1–3 or 1–4, respectively, and 4 doses of mitoxantrone from days 2–5.

Reference
Hiddemann, W. *et al. 4th International Conference on Malignant Lymphoma, June 6–9, 1990,* Lugano, Switzerland.

IMVP-16 (IME)

Ifosfamide*	1 g/m^2 in 1000 ml dextrose water	IV	over 1 h on days 1–5
MTX	30 mg/m^2	IM	days 3–10
Etoposide	100 mg/m^2 in 1000 ml normal saline	IV	over 2 h on days 1–3

*MESNA is given as in MIME or DICE

References
Cabanillas, F. *et al.* (1983). *Am. J. Med.* **74,** 382–388.
Cabanillas, F. *et al.* (1982). *Blood,* **60,** 693–697

MIME

Methyl GAG*	500 mg/m^2	IV	days 1 and 14
Ifosfamide	1000 mg/m^2	IV	days 1–5
MTX	30 mg/m^2	IV	day 3
Etoposide†	100 mg/m^2	IV	day 1–3

*Methyl GAG on day 14 omitted if mucositis present.
†Infused over a minimum of 1 h.

MESNA and Hydration are recommended to prevent hemorrhagic cystitis from ifosfamide. It is given after first infusion of ifosfamide at 900 mg/m^2/24 h (i.e. 300 mg/m^2 MESNA/normal saline). Continue MESNA infusion for 12 h after last dose of ifosfamide.

In addition 200 mg/m^2 MESNA is given in 50 ml of N/S by rapid infusion over 5–10 m, 1 h prior to each ifosamide infusion during days 1–4.

No treatment given from days 6 or 15–21 and/or 28.

Reference
Hagemeister, F.B. *et al.* (1987). *J. Clin. Oncol.* **5,** 556–561.

MINE*

MESNA	1·3 g/m^2/day and 500 g	IV PO	for 3 days 4 h after each ifosfamide dose is given
Ifosfamide	1·33 g/m^2/day	IV	days 1–3
Novantrone	8 mg/m^2	IV	day 1
Etoposide	65 mg/m^2	IV	days 1–3

No treatment from days 5–21.
*MINE is given until maximum response (if CR = 6 cycles); followed by consolidation with three courses of ESAP.

Reference
Cabanillas, F., Rodriguez, M.A. *et al. 4th International Conference on Malignant Lymphoma, June 6–9, 1990.* Lugano, Switzerland.

MIV

Mitoxantrone	10 mg/m^2	IV	day 1
Ifosfamide*	1500 mg/m^2	IV	days 1–3
VP-16	150 mg/m^2	IV	days 1–3

No treatment on days 4–21.
*MESNA given as in MINE.

Reference
Herbrecht, R. *et al. 4th International Conference on Malignant Lymphoma, June 6–9, 1990,* Lugano, Switzerland.

VP-I-P*

VP-16	75 mg/m^2	IV	days 1–5
Ifosfamide	1·2 g/m^2	IV	days 1–4 (max dose 1·75 g)
Cis-platinum	20 mg/m^2	IV	days 1–5

MESNA 120 mg/m^2 IV bolus is given prior to ifosfamide and 400 mg/m^2/day IV infusion is given for 5 ½ days continuing for 36 h after the last dose of ifosfamide.

Reference

Loehrer, P.J., Einhorn, L.H. *et al.* (1986). *J. Clin. Oncol.* **4,** 528–536.
Loehrer, P.J., Lauer, R. *et al.* (1988). *Ann. Int. Med.* **109,** 540–545.
Haim, N. *et al.* (1990). *Ann. Oncol.* **1,** 4 (Abstract p1:12).

*As for refractory germ cell tumor; has been used with some success with transient response in refractory lymphoma starting with 75 % of the dose above.

UNDIFFERENTIATED/LYMPHOBLASTIC OR BURKITT'S LYMPHOMA

A number of different protocols are available, some of them similar to regimens used to treat acute lymphoblastic leukemia. One of these proposed in the USA is given here.

Cycle 1

Cyclophosphamide	1200 mg/m^2	IV	day 1
MTX	300 mg/m^2	IV	in first hour on days 10–12
	and 60 mg/m^2/h for the next 2–42 h (total 2·7 g/m^2)	IV	Followed by Leucovorin rescue
Ara-C	30 mg/m^2	IT	days 1, 2, 3 and 6
MTX	12·5 mg	IT	day 10

Cycles 2 and 3

Vincristine	1·4 mg/m^2	IV	day 1
Adriamycin	40 mg/m^2	IV	day 1
Cyclophosphamide	1200 mg/m^2	IV	day 1
Prednisone	40 mg/m^2	PO	days 1–5
MTX	IV as in cycle 1		days 10–12

Ara C and MTX IT as in cycle 1 (days 1–3 and on day 10)

Cycles 4–6

IV as above in cycles 2 and 3.
IT Ara-C 30 mg/m^2, on days 1 and 10.

Cycles 7–15

IV as above in cycles 4–6.
IV MTX as above on days 13–15.

Table 8. Undifferentiated lymphoma or lymphoblastic lymphoma

Cycles commence as soon as granulocyte count is above 1500 /mm^3 (or day 28 for cycles 7–15). Total of 15 cycles given almost every 28–30 days.

Cycle 1

Day	1	2	3	4	5	6	7	8	9	10	11	12	13	14	15
Cyclophosphamide 1200 mg/m^2 (IV)	↑														
MTX 300 mg/m^2 1st h (IV) 60 mg/m^2, 2–42h (IV) + leucovorin rescue										↑	↑	↑			
Vincristine 1·4 mg/m^2 (IV)															
Adriamycin 40 mg/m^2 (IV)															
Prednisone 40 mg/m^2 (PO)															
MTX 12·5 mg/m^2 (IT) (max 12·5 mg)										↑					
Ara-C 30 mg/m^2 (IT)	↑	↑	↑			↑									

Cycles 2–3

Day	1	2	3	4	5	6	7	8	9	10	11	12	13	14	15
Cyclophosphamide 1200 mg/m^2 (IV)	↑														
MTX 300 mg/m^2 1st h (IV) 60 mg/m^2, 2–42h (IV) + leucovorin rescue										↑	↑	↑			
Vincristine 1·4 mg/m^2 (IV)	↑														
Adriamycin 40 mg/m^2 (IV)	↑														
Prednisone 40 mg/m^2 (PO)	PO	PO	PO	PO	PO										
MTX 12·5 mg/m^2 (IT) (max 12·5 mg)			↑							↑					
Ara-C 30 mg/m^2 (IT)	↑	↑													

Cycles 4–6

Day	1	2	3	4	5	6	7	8	9	10	11	12	13	14	15
Cyclophosphamide 1200 mg/m^2 (IV)	↑														
MTX 300 mg/m^2 1st h (IV) 60 mg/m^2, 2–42h (IV) + leucovorin rescue										↑	↑	↑			
Vincristine 1·4 mg/m^2 (IV)	↑														
Adriamycin 40 mg/m^2 (IV)	↑														
Prednisone 40 mg/m^2 (PO)	PO	PO	PO	PO	PO										
MTX 12·5 mg/m^2 (IT) (max 12·5 mg)										↑					
Ara-C 30 mg/m^2 (IT)	↑														

Cycles 7–15

Day	1	2	3	4	5	6	7	8	9	10	11	12	13	14	15
Cyclophosphamide 1200 mg/m^2 (IV)	↑														
MTX 300 mg/m^2 1st h (IV) 60 mg/m^2, 2–42h (IV) + leucovorin rescue													↑	↑	↑
Vincristine 1·4 mg/m^2 (IV)	↑														
Adriamycin 40 mg/m^2 (IV)	↑														
Prednisone 40 mg/m^2 (PO)	PO	PO	PO	PO	PO										
MTX 12·5 mg/m^2 (IT) (max 12·5 mg)															
Ara-C 30 mg/m^2 (IT)															

Reference

Magrath, I.T. *et al.* (1984). *Blood* **63,** 1102–1111.

A total of *15 cycles* are given; each cycle is given every 28–30 days or when the granulocyte count is above $1{\cdot}5\times10^9$/l (see Table 8).

Reference

Magrath, I.T. *et al.* (1984). *Blood* **63,** 1102–1111.

LYMPHOBLASTIC LYMPHOMA

This representative regimen from the USA, is given as an example of this type of therapy. This regimen includes 1 month of induction, 1 month of CNS prophylaxis, 3 months of consolidation and 7 months of maintenance therapy, summarized below.

Cyclophosphamide, 400 mg/m^2 PO for 3 days on weeks 1, 4, 9, 12, 15 and 18.

Adriamycin 50 mg/m^2 IV on weeks 1, 4, 9, 12, 15 and 18.

Vincristine 2 mg/m^2 IV on weeks 1, 6, 9, 12, 14 and 18.

Prednisone 40 mg/m^2 PO daily for 6 weeks (tapered off); then for 5 days on weeks 9, 12, 15 and 18.

L-Asparaginase 6000 units/m^2 IM (maximum 10 000 units) for five doses at the beginning of CNS therapy.

CNS prophylaxis includes whole brain irradiation (2400 cGy in 12 fractions) and IT MTX (12 mg for each of 6 doses) given between weeks 4–9.

Maintenance therapy consists of 30 mg/m^2 MTX PO weekly and 6-MP (75 mg/m^2 PO per day) on weeks 23–52.

Similar regimen

Cyclophosphamide	400 mg/m^2	PO	3 days during weeks 1, 4, 9, 12, 15 and 18.
Doxorubicin	50 mg/m^2	IV	day 1 during weeks 1, 4, 9, 12, 15 and 18.
Vincristine	2 mg/m^2		during weeks 1, 2, 3, 4, 5, 6, 9, 12, 15, and 18
Prednisone	40 mg/day	PO	daily for first 4 weeks, tapered to 5 days from weeks 5–9; further tapering 10–22; 23–52 weeks (stop).
L-Asparaginase	6000 i.u./m^2	IM	5 doses for 9 weeks
MTX	IT prophylaxis 12 mg × 6 doses		weeks 4–9
Maintenance			
6-MP	75 mg/m^2/day	PO	weeks 23–52
MTX	30 mg/m^2/day	PO	weeks 23–52
Cranial Irradiation	2400 CGY		weeks 5–9

References

Casciato, D.A. and Lowitz, B.B. (1989). *Manual of Clinical Oncology,* 2nd edn, p. 336. Boston, Mass.: Little, Brown & Co.

Coleman *et al.* (1986). *J. Clin. Oncol.* **4,** 1628–1637.

Another alternative regimen

APO

Induction (days 1–29)

Adriamycin	75 mg/m^2	days 1 and 22
Prednisone	40 mg/m^2	days 1–29
Oncovin	1·5 mg/m^2	days 1, 8, 15, 22 and 29

Consolidation (weeks 6–8)

Adriamycin	30 mg/m^2		day 1
Prednisone	120 mg/m^2		days 1–5
Oncovin	2 mg/m^2 (maximum 2 mg)		day 1
6-MP	225 mg/m^2	PO	days 1–5

and L-asparaginase 56 000 i.u./m^2 for patients younger than 6 years or 28 000 i.u./m^2 for patients older than 6 years, IM or IV for five doses days 1–5

Preventive CNS

MTX 12 mg/m^2 IT (maximum 12 mg) for 5 doses, and cranial irradiation 2400 rad in 13 fractions over 17 days.

Maintenance (weeks 12–104)

Adriamycin, Oncovin, prednisone and 6-MP are given in the same regimen as for consolidation every 3 weeks to a cumulative dose of 450 mg/m^2 of Adriamycin, then MTX is substituted (7·5 mg/m^2/day) for 5 days, IV on day 1, IM on days 2–5 instead of Adriamycin.

Alternative regimen for BURKITT'S LYMPHOMA (USA)

Induction Therapy

A.	Cyclophosphamide	1g/m^2	IV	day 1
	Vincristine	1·5mg/m^2	IV	day 1
	Ara C	40mg/m^2	IT	days 1–3
B.	Vincristine	1·5mg/m^2	IV	day 8
	Methotrexate**	3g/m^2	IV	day 8
	Methotrexate	12 mg	IT	day 8, followed by
	Leucovorin, 24 hours later		IV	(as in other regimens)
C.†	Cyclophosphamide	1g/m^2	IV	day 15
	Vincristine	1·5mg/m^2	IV	day 15
	Ara C***	3g/m^2	IV	days 15–18
	Ara C	40mg/m^2	IT	day 15

** (given as for high dose Methotrexate regimens)
*** (given over 3 hours and every 12 hours for 4 days; 8 doses)

†provided platelet count is greater than 100 × 10^9/liter and neutrophil count > 200 and rising; otherwise delay.

D.	Vincristine	1·5mg/m^2	IV	day 22
E.	Methotrexate	3g/m^2	IV	day 36
	followed by Leucovorin as in (B)			
	Methotrexate	12mg/m^2	IT	day 36

Consolidation Therapy

A.	Cyclophosphamide	1g/m^2	IV	day 43
	Vincristine	1·5mg/m^2	IV	day 43
	Ara-C	3g/m^2	IV	days 43–45
	(given over 3 hours and every 12 hours for 3 days; 6 doses)			
	Ara-C	40mg/m^2	IT	day 43
B.	Methotrexate	3g/m^2	IV	day 57
	(as on days 8 and 36) followed by Leucovorin on day 58 for 3 days.			
	Methotrexate	12mg	IT	day 57

Reference

As used at N.I.H., USA.

MULTIPLE MYELOMA

SINGLE AGENTS OR TWO DRUG REGIMENS

Alkeran (melphalan) as intermittent or continuous daily oral therapy.

0·25 mg/kg for a few days followed by 0·1 mg/kg/day for a further 7–10 days or a loading dose of 0·1 mg/kg/day for 14 days with rest periods of 3–4 weeks or, alternatively, 2–6 mg/day with adjustments to be made depending on the blood counts. This can be used together with or without a varying dose of prednisone 20–40 mg/day for as long as the intermittent alkeran is used.

Methylprednisolone
1·5 g/day PO for 1–5 days

Cyclophosphamide and Prednisone

Cyclosphamide	300 mg/m^2	IV	weekly
Prednisone	40 mg/m^2	PO	6–8 weeks

or

Cyclosphamide	1·2 g/m^2	IV	days 1–4
Prednisone	90 mg/m^2	PO	days 1–4

References

Alexanian, R. *et al.* (1983). *Blood* **62,** 572–577.
Bergsagel, D.F. *et al.* (1972). *Canad. Med. Assoc. J.* **107,** 851–855.
Oken, M.M. (1986). *Med. Clin. North Am.* **68 (3),** 300–309.
Salmon, S.E. *et al.* (1983). *J. Clin. Oncol.* **1,** 453–461.
Barlogie, B. *et al.* (1986). *Blood* **67,** 1248–1301.
Mandelli, F. *et al.* (1990). *New Engl. J. Med.* **372,** 1430–1435.

High-dose alkeran (melphalan) (autologous BMT)
If glomerular filtration greater than 40 ml/min.
40 mg/m^2 IV or up to 200 mg/m^2 IV depending on whether autologous BMT is done or not. Patients may be primed first with 400 mg/m^2 IV

cyclophosphamide given 1 week before melphalan with forced saline diuresis. Prophylactic antifungal and antibacterial drugs are given.

Reference

Selby, P., McElwain, T.J. *et al.* (1987). *Brit. J. Haematol.* **66,** 55–62.
Gore *et al.* (1989). *Lancet* **14,** 879–882.
Mandelli, F. *et al.* (1990). *New Engl. J. Med.* **322,** 1430–1435.

Alpha-Interferon

For use see combined regimens (p 125).

COMBINED REGIMENS

ABCP

Adriamycin	20 mg/m^2	IV	day 1 or 2
BCNU	50 mg/m^2	IV	day 1
Cyclophosphamide	200 mg/m^2	IV	day 1
Prednisone	60 mg/m^2	PO	days 1–5

No treatment given from days 6–21.

Reference

Presant, C.A. and Klahr, C. (1978). *Cancer* **42,** 1222–1227.

CAP–BAP

CAP

Cyclophosphamdide	400 mg/m^2	IV	day 1
Adriamycin	30 mg/m^2	IV	day 1
Prednisone	0.6 mg/m^2	PO	days 1–7

No treatment given between days 8–21.

BAP

BCNU	75 mg/m^2	IV	days 1 and 22
Adriamycin	30 mg/m^2	IV	day 1
Prednisone	0·6 mg/m2	PO	days 1–7

No treatment from days 22–35.

Reference
Kyle, R.A. *et al.* (1982). *Cancer Treat. Rep.* **66,** 451–456.

Recombinant Alpha-Interferon

α-Interferon can be added during the *induction and maintenance phase* of some of the above described protocols as 3–6 $\times 10^6$ i.u./m^2/day by SC/IM injection daily.

or

3–6 $\times 10^6$ i.u./m^2/day as SC/IM 3 times weekly during the maintenance phase after plateau phase of the myeloma is reached.

References
Oken, M.M., Kyle, R.A. *et al.* (1988). *Proc. Am. Soc. Clin. Oncol.* **7,** 868a.
Oken, M.M. *et al.* (1990). *Leukemia and Lymphoma* **1,** 95–100.
Alexanian, R. *et al.* (1982). *Clin. Haematol.* **11,** 211–220.
Mandelli, F. *et al.* (1990). *New Engl. J. Med.* **322,** 1430–1435.

M2 REGIMEN (See VBMCP)

VAD

Vincristine	0·4 mg/day continuous infusion	IV	days 1–4
Adriamycin	9 mg/m^2/day continuous infusion	IV	days 1–4
Dexamethasone	40 mg/day	IV	days 1–4 9–12 17–20

No treatment is given from days 21–28.

References

Barlogie, B. *et al.* (1984). *New Engl. J. Med.* **310,** 1353–1356.
Scheehan, T. *et al.* (1986). *Scand. J. Haematol.* **37,** 425–428.
Samson, D. *et al.* (1989). *Lancet* **14,** 882–885.
Alexanian, R. *et al.* (1990). *Am. J. Hematol.* **33,** 86–89.

VAMP

As for VAD (above) with methylprednisolone given at 1·5 g/day PO or IV from days 1–5 instead of dexamethasone.

No treatment given from days 6–21.
This regimen is continued until partial remission (PR) or complete remission (CR) is achieved (up to 11 cycles; median 5).

References

Forgeson, G.V. *et al.* (1988). *Brit. J. Cancer* **58,** 469–473.
Gore, M.E. *et al* (1989). *Lancet,* **14,** 879–881.

VBAP

Vincristine	1 mg	IV	day 1
BCNU	30 mg/M^2	IV	day 1
Adriamycin	30 mg/m^2	IV	day 1
Prednisone	100 mg	PO	days 1 – 4

No treatment given from days 5 – 21.

References

Bonnet, J. et al. (1982). *Cancer Treat. Rep.* **66,** 1267–1271.
Salmon, S.E. *et al.* (1983). *J. Clin. Oncol.* **1,** 453–461.

M2 Regimen* or VBMCP

Vincristine	0.03 mg/kg	IV	day 1 or 21
BCNU	0·5 mg/kg	IV	day 1
Mephalan	0·25 mg/kg	PO	days 1–10
Cyclophosphamide	10 mg/kg	IV	day 1
Prednisone	1 mg/kg	PO	days 1–7
	0·5 mg/kg	PO	days 8–14
	0·3 mg/kg	PO	days 15–21

No treatment given on days 22–35.
If there is response, continue for at least 12 cycles.

References

*Case, C.D., Lee, B.J. *et al.* (1977). *Am. J. Med.* **63,** 897–903.
Oken, M.M. *et al.* (1984). *Proc. Assoc.* **3,** 270.
Mandelli, F. *et al.* (1990). *New Engl. J. Med.* **322,** 1430–1434.

VCAD–VAD

Vincristine	0·4 mg/day continuous infusion	IV	days 1–4
Adriamycin	7 mg/m^2/day continuous infusion	IV	days 1–4
Cyclophosphamide	120 mg/m^2/day	PO	days 1–4
Dexamethasone as in VAD	40 mg/day	IV	days 1–4, 9–12, 17–20

No treatment given from days 4–28.

Followed by **VAD** as on page 125.

No treatment given from day 21–28.

Reference

Alexanian, R. *et al.* (1990). *Am. J. Hematol.* **33,** 86–89.

VCAP

Vincristine	1·5 mg/m^2	IV	day 1
Cyclophosphamide	125 mg/m^2	IV or PO	days 1–4
Adriamycin	30 mg/m^2	IV	day 1
Prednisone	60 mg/m^2	PO	days 1–4

No treatment given from days 5–21.

References

Alexanian, R. and Dreicer, R. (1984). *Cancer* **53,** 583–588.
Salmon *et al.* (1983). *J. Clin. Oncol.* **1,** 453–461.

ACUTE LEUKEMIA

For obvious reasons *all* existing chemotherapy regimens and trials are *not* listed in this chapter. These protocols vary from country to country as do the results of therapy. Differences of opinion exist with some controversy arising from the evaluation of these results. Accordingly, only representative and frequently used regimens have been included.

The advent of autologous and allogeneic BMTs has also altered the concepts of induction, consolidation, maintenance and intensification for acute leukemias. Furthermore there are still differences in opinion as to who should be transplanted and when. Specific protocols are *not* proposed here and guidelines for transplantation are *not* given. Details of *some* of the induction and maintenance schedules used in recent years are provided and I am sure some excellent local combination regimens have been omitted, but without intent or injury.

ACUTE NON-LYMPHOBLASTIC LEUKEMIA

ADOAP (See listed under ROAP)

COAP

Cyclophosphamide	100 mg/m^2	IV	days 1–5
Oncovin	2 mg	IV	day 1
Ara-C	200 mg/m^2	IV	continuous on days 1–5
Prednisone	25 mg q.i.d.	PO	days 1–5

Alternative COAP regimens

Cyclophosphamide	600 mg/m^2	IV	day 1
Oncovin	1·5 mg/m^2	IV	day 1
Ara-C	100 mg/m^2	IV	continuous on days 1–5
Prednisolone	60 mg/m^2	PO	days 1–5

Reference

Coltman, C.A. *et al.* (1978). *Arch. Int. Med.* 137, 1342–1348.
Cassileth, P.A. and Katz, M.E. (1977). *Cancer Chemotherapy Rep.* **61,** 1441–1445.
Keating, M.J. (1982). *Cancer Treatment and Research,* **5,** 237–263. Edited by C. Bloomfield. Boston: Martinus Nijhoff Publishers.

DAT

Daunorubicin	45 mg/m^2	IV	days 1–3
Ara-C	100 mg/m^2	IV	q. 12 h or by continuous infusion on days 1–7 (10).
6-TG	100 mg/m^2	PO	q. 12 h days 1–7

No treatment given from days 7 (10)–21 (28).

Lately 6-TG has been dropped from this regimen. Some authors have given the above combination as a 7+3 or 10+3 combination, while others have given higher doses over short time periods.

e.g.

Daunorubicin	50 mg/m^2	IV	days 1–3
Ara-C	25 mg/m^2	IV bolus	followed by 160 mg/m^2 continuously on days 1–5
6-TG	100 mg/m^2		q. 12 h days 1–5.

No treatment on days 6–21.

References
Foon, K.A. and, Gale R.P. (1987). *Blood* **59,** 1551.
Foon, K.A. and Gales, R.P. (1984). *Recent Results Cancer Res.* **93,** 216–239.
Rai, K.R. *et al.* (1981). *Blood* **58,** 1203–1212.
Preisler, H.D. *et al.* (1979). *Blood,* **53,** 455–464.
Yates, J. *et al.* (1982). *Blood* **60,** 4554–462.
Rees, J.K.H. and Hayhoe, F.G.J. (1984). *Proc. ASCO* **3,** 190.
Lewis, J.P. (1984). *Cancer Treatment Rev.* **12.** 133–143.
Arlin, Z. *et al.* (1979). *Proc. Am. Assoc. Canc. Res.* **20,** 112.

DOAP

As in COAP but *daunorubicin* 60 mg/m^2 IV on day 1 instead of cyclophosphamide.

Epirubicin and Ara-C

Epirubicin	45 mg/m$_2$	IV	days 1–3
Ara-C	200 mg/m$_2$	IV	days 1–7

Some have added the following to the above:

VP–16	150 mg/m^2	IV	over 1 h days 1–3
Cyclophosphamide	100 mg/m$_2$	IV	days 1–5

No treatment on days 6–21.

Reference
Jankovic, M. *et al.* (1990). *Leukemia and Lymphoma* **1,** 203–208.

GAC (using methyl GAG)*

Methyl GAG	150 mg/m^2	IV	days 1, 3 and 5
Ara-C	100 mg/m^2	IV or SC	days 1–5
Cyclophosphamide	600 mg/m^2	IV	day 1
or			
Repeated maintenance			
6-MP	25 mg/kg/day	PO	
MTX	15 mg/m^2	PO or IM	weekly
and			
Daunomycin	30 mg/m^2	IV	days 1 and 2
Methyl GAG	250 mg/m^2	IV	days 3, 5 and 8 during months 2, 4, 8, 12, 18, 24 and 30

*This is just one of the regimens used.

References

Bernard, J. *et al.* (1973). *Blood* **41,** 489–496.
Kantarajian, H.M. *et al.* (1986). *Am. J. Med.* **80,** 789.

IAE

Idarubicin	8 mg/m^2	IV	days 1–5
Ara-C	200 mg/m^2	IV	continuous infusion days 1–5
Etoposide	150 mg/m^2	IV	in a 2 h infusion days 1–3

No treatment on days 6–21.

Course given at the same dosage but only 2 days idarubicin. If CR achieved use four courses of post-remission intensification using:

Idarubicin	10 mg/m^2	IV	day 1
Ara-C	60 mg/m^2	SC	q. 8 h days 1–5
6-TG	70 mg/m^2	PO	q. 8 h days 1–5

Subsequent escalation of Ara-C (80 mg/m^2, 110 mg/m^2, 150 mg/m^2).

Reference

Carella, A.M. *et al.* (1987). *In Mandelli, Idarubicin in the Treatment of Acute Leukemia. Exc. Medica.* Amsterdam. p 26–36.

Idarubicin and Ara-C

Similar regimen as for DAT but *idarubicin* replaces daunorubicin

Idarubicin	12 or 13 mg/m^2 IV	days 1–3
Ara-C	100 mg/m^2 IV	continuous infusion days 1–7
	or 200 mg/m^2	continuous infusion days 1–5

References

Berman, E. *et al.* (1989). *Sem. Oncol.* **16,** 30–34.
Vogler, W.R. *et al.* (1989). *Sem. Oncol.* **16,** 21–24.
Wiernik, P. *et al.* (1989). *Sem. Oncol.* **16,** 25–29.

Alternatively
Idarubicin has also been used 20mg/m^2 PO. (Reference: Bezwoda, W.R. and Dansey, R.D. (1990). *Leukemia and Lymphoma* **1,** 221–225).
A loading dose of 25 mg/m^2 IV bolus Ara-C has been used (Reference: Petti, M. *et al.* (1989). *Sem. Oncol.* **16,** 10–15).

***m*-AMSA and Ara-C**

The above DAT regimen may be used with *m*-AMSA IV 190 mg/m^2 on days 1–3, replacing daunorubicin.

Reference

Louie, A.C. and Issel, F. (1985). *J. Clin. Oncol.* **3,** 562.
Arlin, Z.A. et al. (1980). *Cancer Res.* **40,** 3304–3306.

Mitoxantrone and Ara-C

Same regimen as for DAT but 6–12 mg/m^2 *Mitoxantrone* given IV on days 1–3 or 1–5 instead of daunorubicin.

References

Prentice, H.G. *et al.* (1985). *Inv. New Drugs* **3,** 207–212.
Shenkenberg, T.D. and Von Hoff, D.D. (1986). *Ann. Int. Med.* **105,** 67.
Arlin, Z.A. (1990). *Leukemia and Lymphoma* **1,** 301–305.
Arlin, Z.A. (1988). *Proc. ASCO* **7,** 186.

OAP

This is given *without* cyclophosphamide, increasing Ara-C to 200 mg/m^2 continuous IV infusion on days 1–5.

POMP

Prednisone	16 mg/m^2	PO	days 1–5
Oncovin	2 mg	IV	day 1
MTX	7·5 mg/m^2	IV	days 1–5
6-MP (purinethol)	500 mg/m^2	IV	days 1–5

No treatment from days 6–14.
May be used as intensification after induction and consolidation or as maintenance as decribed in Spiers (1972).

References

Spiers. A.S.D. (1972). *Clinics Hemat.* **1,** 127–164.
Wiernik, P.H. and Serpick, A.A. (1972). *Canc. Res.* **32,** 2023–2026.
Preisler, H.D. (1982). *Cancer Treatment and Research,* vol. 5, pp. 155–197. Edited by C. Bloomfield. Boston: Martinus Nijhoff Publishers.
Keating, M.J. (1982). *Cancer Treatment and Research,* vol. 5, pp. 237–263. Edited by C. Bloomfield. Boston: Martinus Nijhoff Publishers.

ROAP

Ara-C	55–70 mg/m^2	IV	continuous on days 1–7
Oncovin	2·0 mg/m^2	IV	day 1
Prednisone	25 mg q.i.d.	PO	days 1–5
Rubidazone	150–200 mg/m^2	IV	day 1

No treatment given from days 7–21.

ADOAP

As for ROAP but *Adriamycin 40 mg/m^2* IV on day 1 instead of rubidazone.

No treatment given from days 7–21.
Used in the elderly.

References

Keating, M.J. *et al.* (1981). *Blood* **58,** 584–591.
Peterson, B.A. (1982). *Cancer Treatment and Research* **5,** 199–236. Edited by C. Bloomfield, Boston: Martinus Nijhoff Publishers.

VAPA

Vincristine	1·5 mg/m^2	IV	days 1 and 5
Adriamycin	30 mg/m^2	IV	days 1–3
Prednisolone	40 mg/m^2	IV	q. 12 h on days 1–7
Ara-C	100 mg/m^2	IV	q. 12 h on days 1–7

No treatment given on days 6–21. If CR is obtained, a second course is given over 5 days only (Ara-C, days 1–5). If no CR but good PR give 7 days cycle.

If CR is achieved, sequential intensive maintenance is given every 3–4 weeks.

Sequence 1 (×4)			
Adriamycin	45 mg/m^2	IV	day 1
Ara-C	200 mg/m^2	IV	continuous on days 1–5
Sequence 2 (×4)			
Adriamycin	30 mg/m^2/day	IV	day 1
Azacytidine	150 mg/m^2/day	IV	days 1–5
Sequence 3 (×4)			
Vincristine	1·5 mg/m^2/day	IV	day 1
Methylprednisolone	800 mg/m^2/day	IV	days 1–5
6-MP	500 mg/m^2 day	IV	days 1–5
MTX	7·5 mg/m^2/day	IV	days 1–5
Sequence 4 (×4)			
Ara-C	200 mg/m^2	IV	continuous on days 1–5

Reference

Weinstein, H.J. *et al.* (1983). *Blood* **62 (2),** 315.
Weinstein, H.J. *et al.* (1980). *New Engl. J. Med.* **303,** 473–478.

An example of an alternating induction regimen (random example)

Cycle 1			
Ara-C	100 mg/m^2	IV	continuous on days 1–7
Daunomycin	45 mg/m^2	IV	day 1–3
Cycle 2	as above or for 5 days		
Cycle 3			
Ara-C (Intermediate-dose)	500–1000 mg/m^2	IV	q. 12 h on days 1–5
Cycle 4			
Mitoxantrone	12 mg/m^2	IV	days 1–3
5-Azacytidine	1500–200 mg/m^2	IV	continuous on days 1–5
Etoposide	100 mg/m^2	IV	days 1–5

*This cyclic alternating regimen for the induction of leukemia is just a single example of the type of regimens employed utilizing different combinations for induction of remission.

ACUTE PROMYELOCYTIC LEUKEMIA

Some have suggested *a different induction regimen* based on ***daunomycin*** alone, followed by varying consolidation or maintenance and intensification regimens*.

Daunomycin 2 mg/kg/day for 46 days and appropriate therapy for disseminated intravascular coagulation (DIC) including *heparin* IV infusion, 1–1·5 mg/kg/day, fresh frozen plasma and platelet transfusions. Others have used the regular induction regimens including ***daunomycin/m-AMSA, Ara-C*** and ***6-TG.***

Remission is usually consolidated and maintained with rotational combination chemotherapy using alternating POMP, COAP and GAC or 7 day cycles of DAT (using Adriamycin or lower dose daunomycin) or oral therapy with 6-MP, MTX and IV methyl GAG.

References
*Bernard, J. *et al.* (1973). *Blood* **41,** 489–496.
Sanz, M.A. *et al.* (1988). *Cancer* **61,** 7–13.
Sanz, G.F. *et al.* (1990). *Leukemia and Lymphoma* **2,** 85–92.

REGIMENS FOR RELAPSED OR REFRACTORY LEUKEMIA

Some of these may well have been introduced as part of frontline primary induction therapy by some groups and used in some trials by now.

DAC (on page 142)

As for DA + CCNU, 200 mg/m^2 PO on day 1.

If patients in CR a single course of intensive consolidation is given with:

Mitoxantrone	15 mg/m^2	IV	days 1 and 2
Ara-C	2 g/m^2	IV	q. 12 h days 1–4
Etoposide	100 mg/m^2	IV	days 1 and 2

This regimen can be followed by autologous or allogeneic BMT. If not, two additional cycles of consolidation are given with mitoxantrone, Ara-C and etoposide as above.

References
Barrett, J.P. *et al.* (1991). *Leukemia and Lymphoma* **3**: 139–145.
Vernant, J.P. *et al.* (1987). *4th International. Symposium on Therapy of Acute Leukemias. Abstracts, p. 260.* Rome, Italy.

HiDAC and epirubicin/idarubicin/L-asparaginase/ *m*-AMSA/mitoxantrone

*High-dose Ara-C (HiDAC)	3 g/m^2	IV	q.12 h days 1–4
or			
Intermediate-dose Ara-C (IDAC)	0·5–1·5 g/m^2	IV	q. 12 h days 1–4

*Given within 3–6 h for 4 days but schedules vary and some use it for up to 6 days.

and			
Epirubicin	30 mg/m^2		days 1–3
or			
Idarubicin	12 mg/m^2		days 1–3
or			
L-Asparaginase	6000 i.u./m^2	IM	given 3 h after the last dose of Ara-C
or			
m-AMSA	190–200 mg/m^2	IV	days 1–3
or			
Mitoxantrone	6–12 mg/m^2	IV	days 1–3

*** Sequential High-Dose Ara-C and L-Asparaginase (HiDAC ASNASE)**

Time	Drug		Dose
0–3 h	Ara-C	(IV)	3 g/m^2
12–15 h	Ara-C	(IV)	3 g/m^2
24–27 h	Ara-C	(IV)	3 g/m^2
36–39 h	Ara-C	(IV)	3 g/m^2
42 h	L-Asparaginase	(IM)	6000 i.u./m^2

Course repeated if possible after 8–10 days.

Reference

*Capizzi *et al.* (1984). *Blood* **63,** 694.

Idarubicin + Ara-C

These are just a few examples of this regimen. For further variations see the list of references below.

Idarubicin	12 mg/m^2	IV	days 1–3
Ara-C	120 mg/m^2	bd	days 4–10

Idarubicin	8 mg/m^2	IV	days 1–5
Ara-C	1 g/m^2	bd	days 1–3

Idarubicin	12 mg/m^2	IV	days 1–3
Ara-C	600 mg/m^2	bd	days 1–6

References

Willemze, R. *et al.* (1982). *Scand. J. Haematol.* **29,** 141–146
Amadori, S. *et al.* (1984). *Leuk. Res.* **8,** 729–735.
Cantin, G. and Brennan, J.K. (1984). *Am. J. Hematol.* **16,** 59–66.
*Capizzi, R.L. *et al.* (1984). *Blood* **63,** 694.
Hines, J.D. *et al.* (1984). *J. Cliin. Oncol.* **2,** 545–549.
Arlin Z.A. *et al.* (1985). Cancer Treat. Rep. **69,** 1001–1002.
Marcus, D.E. *et al.* (1985). *Lancet* **1,** 1384.
Zittoun, R. *et al.* (1985). *Cancer Treat. Rep.* **69,** 1447–1448.
Fulle, H.H. and Hellriegel K.P. (1986) *Onkologie* **9:** 152–153.
Vogler, W.R. *et al.* (1986). *Cancer Treat. Rep.* **70,** 455–459.
Brito-Babapulle, F. *et al.* (1987). *Cancer Treat. Rep.* **71,** 161–163.
Decker, R.W. *et al.* (1987). *Cancer Treat. Rep.* **71,** 881–882.
Hiddemann, W. *et al.* (1987). *Semi. Oncol.* **14,** 73–77.
Hiddemann, W. *et al.* (1987). *Blood* **69,** 744–749.
Lambertenghi-Deliliers G. et al. (1987) *Eur. J. Clin. Oncol.* 23: 1041–1045.
Capizzi, R.L. *et al.* (1988). *J. Clin. Oncol.* **6,** 499–508.
Berman E. et al. (1989) *Cancer Res.* **49:** 477–481.
Carella A.M. et al. (1989) *Eur. J. Haematol.* **43:** 309–313.
Harousseau J.L. et al. (1989) *J. Clin. Oncol.* **7:** 45–49.
Leone G. et al. (1989) *Haematologica,* **74:** 57–61.

Hiddemann, W. and Büchner, T. (1990). *Blut* **60,** 163–171.
Jancovic, M. *et al.* (1990). *Leukemia and Lymphoma* **1,** 203–208.

VP-16 and 5-Azacytidine

VP-16	250 mg/m^2	IV	days 1–3
5-Azacytidine	300 mg/m^2	IV	days 4–5

No treatment from days 6–14 (21)

Reference

Hakami, N. *et al.* (1987). *J. Clin. Oncol.* **5,** 1022–1025.

***m*-AMSA or Mitoxantrone** can be used instead of 5-azacytidine as page 139.

References

Hiddemann, W. *et al.* (1985). *Onkologie* **8,** 181–184.
Letendre, L. *et al.* (1985). *Med. Ped. Oncol.* **13,** 232–234.
Tschopp, L. *et al.* (1986). *J. Clin. Oncol.* **4,** 318–324.
Ho, W. *et al.* (1988). *J. Clin. Oncol.* **6,** 213–217.
Hiddemann, W. and Büchner, T. (1990). *Blut* **60,** 163–171.

High-dose VP-16 + IDAC

VP-16	200 mg/m^2	IV	days 1–4 in 1 h infusion daily
Ara-C	500 mg–3 g/m^2	IV	12 h in a 1h infusion for 12 doses on days 1–6

No treatment from days 7–21.

References

Chan, H.Y. *et al.* (1987). *Cancer Chemotherapy and Pharmacology* **20,** 265–266.
Freund, M. *et al.* (1987). *Blut* **55,** 215.
Hiddemann, W. and Büchner, (1990). T. *Blut* **60,** 163–171.

Example of a regimen used in a recent current MRC trial for AML

Daunomycin	50 mg/m^2	IV	days 1, 3 and 5
Ara-C	100 mg/m^2	IV	q. 12 h on days 1–10
6-TG	100 mg/m^2	PO	q. 12 h on days 1–10
or			
Etoposide	100 mg/m^2	IV	1 h infusion given on days 1–5 instead of 6-TG

No treatment from day 11–24.
If CR achieved, next cycle is given over 8 days instead of 10.

This is followed by two more cycles:

MACE

m-AMSA	100 mg/m^2		days 1–5
Ara-C	200 mg/m^2	IV	days 1–5
Etoposide	100 mg/m^2	IV	days 1–5

M-IDAC

Mitozantrone	10 mg/m^2	IV	days 1–5
Ara-C	1·0 g/m^2	IV	q. 12 h days 1–3

ANOTHER EXAMPLE OF INDUCTION AND CONSOLIDATION REGIMENS

DA and DAC

Daunorubicin	50 mg/m^2	IV	days 1–3
Ara-C	100 mg/m^2	IV	q. 12 h days 1–7
followed by cycles of:			
Daunorubicin	30 mg/m^2	IV	days 1 and 2
Ara-C	1 g/m^2	IV	q. 12 h on days 1–5

No treatment from days 6–21.

MAZE

m-AMSA	100 mg/m^2	IV	days 1–5
5-Azacytidine	100 mg/m^2	IV	days 1–5
Etoposide	100 mg/m^2	IV	days 1–5

No treatment from days 6–21.
BMT is optional.

ACUTE LYMPHOBLASTIC LEUKEMIA

Only a few examples are given here of the complicated combination chemotherapeutic regimens used currently and in the recent past. For obvious reasons it is impossible to cover all the different regimens used in ALL throughout the world. I include some representative protocols and refer the reader to a list of rcferences which will provide more details and alternative approaches based on the same guidelines outlined here.

L-10 type ALL protocol ("older" protocol)

Vincristine	1·5 mg/m^2	IV	days 1, 8, 15, 22 and 29
Adriamycin	20 mg/m^2	IV	days 18, 19 and 20
Prednisone	60 mg/m^2	PO	days 1–35
MTX	15 mg/m^2	IV	days 42–46 (5 days) 78–82 (5 days) 113–117 (5 days)
MTX	6·25 mg/m^2 or Omaya reservoir	IT	days 1 and 2, 14 and 15 28 and 29, 59–60, 90–91
Ara-C	3·0 mg/kg	IV	q.12 h days 58–65 (8 days) days 93–100 (8 days) days 128–135 (8 days)
Thioguanine	2·5 mg/kg	PO	q.12 h – as for Ara-C
L-Asparaginase	200 i.u./kg	IV	days 135–148 (14 days)
Cyclophosphamide	1200 mg/m^2	IV	day 148

This is followed by a **maintenance** protocol starting after the first **150 days** of induction employing the following:

Vincristine	1·5 mg/m^2	IV	days 1 and 8, 72 and 80
Prednisone	90 mg/m^2	PO	days 1–7, 73–80
Adriamycin	20 mg/m^2	IV	days 14, 15 and 16
6-MP	90 mg/m^2	PO	days 30–58 days 102–130
BCNU	80 mg/m^2	IV	day 86
Cyclophosphamide	800 mg/m^2	IV	day 86
MTX	6·24 mg/m^2	IT	2 injections day 30 and 32, 100 and 102
Dactinomycin	1000 mg/m^2	IV	day 67 and 137

This maintenance scheme of 150 days continued for 24–36 months.

Reference

Schauer, P. *et al.* (1983). *J. Clin. Oncol.* **1**, 462.

ALL Protocol (standard risk)

Induction

L-Asparaginase	6000 i.u./m^2	IM	3 ×/week from day 4, weeks 1, 2, and 3 on days 4–7, 11–14, 18–21
Daunorubicin	45 mg/m^2	IV	days 1 and 2, during week 1
Vincristine	1·5 mg/m^2	IV	Max 3 mg/week; weeks 1–4, days 1, 8, 15 and 22
Prednisone	40 mg/m^2	PO	from week 1–5, days 1–28
MTX	10 mg/m^2	IT	once weekly; on weeks 1, 2, 5 and 6 on days 1, 8, 15 and 29

Bone-marrow examination suggested on day 1 and during week 2 and 3.

Intensification *starting on day 29*

Daunorubicin	45 mg/m^2		days 29 and 30
Ara-C	100 mg/m^2	IV	q. 12 h days 31–33
VP-16	100 mg/m^2	IV	days 31–33
6-TG	80 mg/m^2	PO	days 31 and 33
Vincristine	1·5 mg/m^2		day 29, and during weeks 6, 10, 11 and 12
Prednisone	40 mg/m^2	PO	for 5 days on weeks 8 and 12

Bone-marrow examination suggested on day 29.
Cranial radiotherapy 1800 rads during weeks 9–12.

Maintenance (continuing for 24–36 months) 6-MP 75 mg/m^2/day PO starting on week 8 and continuing throughout maintenance.
MTX 20 mg/m^2/week PO starting on week 12 and continuing throughout maintenance.

Vincristine	1·5 mg/m^2	IV	once per month.
Prednisone	40 mg/m^2	PO	x 5 days each month.

One of the recent European style adult ALL protocols (high-risk)

Phase 1a. Induction

L-Asparaginase	5000 i.u./m^2	IV	days 1–14
Daunorubicin	25 mg/m^2	IV	days 1, 8, 15 and 22
Prednisone	60 mg/m^2	PO	days 1–28

Phase 1b. Induction

Cyclophosphamide	650 mg/m^2	IV	days 28, 42 and 56
Ara-C	75 mg/m^2	IV	4 x week during 4 weeks (day 56)
6-MP	60 mg/m^2	PO	days 28–56
Cranial irradiation			days 28–56
MTX	10 mg/m^2	IT	days 28, 35, 42 and 49

Phase 2. Starting on week 10 (day 70)

Ara-C	75 mg/m^2	IV	for 5 days during weeks 10 and 14
VM-26	60 mg/m^2	IV	for 5 days during weeks 10 and 14

Phase 3a. Starting on week 20

Dexamethasone	10 mg/m^2	PO	per day during weeks 20–24, for 5 weeks
Adriamycin	25 mg/m^2	IV	weekly during weeks 20–23 × 4
Vincristine	1·5 mg/m^2	IV	weekly × 4 as above

Phase 3b. Starting week 24–26

Cyclophosphamide	60 mg/m	IV	single injection in week 24
Ara-C	75 mg/m day	IV	for 4 days in weeks 24 and 25
6-TG	60 mg/m/day	PO	during weeks 24 and 25

Phase 4. (weeks 28–38)
Ara-C as in phase 2 during weeks 28–38
VM-26 as in phase 2 during weeks 28–38

Phase 5. (weeks 38–130)
Oral Maintenance with
6-MP 60 mg/m/day PO
MTX 20 mg/m/week PO or IV

In some low risk ALL protocols, phase 2 (weeks 10–18) and phase 4 (weeks 28–38) are replaced by periods of oral maintenance with 6-MP and MTX, while phase 3 (weeks 20–26) is kept using the drugs listed for phases 3a and 3b.

Another recent regimen used for treating adult ALL

Induction

Vincristine	2 mg/m^2	IV	days 1, 8, 15 and 22
Prednisone	60 mg/m^2	PO	days 1–28
Daunorubicin	45 mg/m^2	IV	days 1–3
L-Asparaginase	4000 i.u./m^2		days 17–28

CNS prophylaxis

MTX	12 mg/m^2	IT	days 1, 8, 15, 22, 29 and 36
Cranial irradiation			1800 rads total in 10 fractions

If patient is in CR - systemic therapy is continued with regimens A and B, given on alternate months for 8 months.

Regimen A

Vincristine	2 mg/m^2	IV	days 1 and 8
Prednisone	60 mg/m^2	PO	days 1–14
L-Asparaginase	10 000 i.u./m^2	IM	days 2, 4, 7, 9, 11 and 14

Regimen B

Etoposide	75 mg/m^2	IV	days 1, 4, 8 and 11
Ara-C	300 mg/m^2	IV	days 1, 4, 8 and 11

Regimen C (given during the 9th month)

MTX	700 mg/m^2	IV	42 h continuous infusion
Leucovorin	15 mg/m^2	IV	q. 6 h x 12 doses starting after MTX infusion

Regimen D (given for 20 months)

MTX	20 mg/m^2	PO	weekly
6-MP	75 mg/m^2	PO	daily

All doses are modified according to tolerance.

Reference

Linker, C.A. et al. (1987). *Blood* **69,** 1242–1248.

FAILURE REGIMENS for ALL

High/intermediate-dose Ara-C

Failure regimens similar to those employed in ANLL based on high- or intermediate-dose **Ara-C +*m*-AMSA,** asparaginase, idarubicin or mitoxantrone may also be attempted when the initial regimen used for induction fails (see ANLL section, page 129).

Slightly different schedules employing combinations of Idarubicin have also been reported.

eg.

Idarubicin	10mg/m^2	weekly
Vincristine	2 mg/m^2	weekly
L-asparaginase	6000 i.u./m^2	day 4 and for alternate days ×9

Reference

Mandelli, F. et al. (1986). *Hematologica,* **71,** 34–38.

SUGGESTED REFERENCES

Chesells, J.M. (1986). *Clin. Haem.* **15**, 727–753.
Clarkson, B. *et al.* (1985). *Sem. Oncol.* **2**, 160–179.
Crist, W. *et al.* (1988). *J. Clin. Oncol.* **6**, 34–43.
Esterhay, R.J. & Wiernik, P.H. (1982). In *Cancer Treatment and Research* vol. 5, pp. 309–349. Edited by C.D. Bloomfield. Boston: Martinus Nijhoff Publishers.

Esterhay, R.J. *et al.* (1982). *Blood* **59**, 334.
Foon, K.A. and Todd R.F. (1986). *Blood* **68**, 1.
Gingrich, R.D. *et al.* (1985). *Cancer Treat. Rep.* **69**, 153.
Gottlieb, A.J. *et al.* (1984). *Blood* **64**, 267–274.
Hoelzer, D. *et al.* (1984). *Blood* **64**, 38–47.
Hoelzer, D. *et al.* (1988). *Blood* **71**, 123–131.
Jacobs, A.D. and Gale, R.P. (1984). *New Engl. J. Med.* **19**, 1219–1231.
Linker, C.A. *et al.* (1987). *Blood* **69**, 1242–1248.
Mauer, A.M. (1980). *J. Am. Soc. Hematol.* **56**, 1–10.
McMillan, A.K. *et al.* (1990). *Leukemia and Lymphoma* **1**, 157–162.
Morra, E. *et al.* (1986). *J. Clin. Oncl.* **4**, 1207.
Neimeyer, C.M. *et al.* (1985). *Sem. Oncol.* **2**, 122–130.
Omura, G.A. *et al.* (1980). *Blood* **55**, 1–10.
Pinkel, D. (1979). *Cancer* **43**, 1128.
Polli, E.E. (1979). *Haematologica* **64**, 119.
Proctor, S.J. *et al.* (1988). *Brit. J. Haem.* **69**, 35–39.
Riehm, H. *et al.* (1980). *Am. J. Ped. Hematol. Oncol.* **2**. 299–306.
Rivera, G. *et al.* (1980). *Cancer* **466**, 1727–1730.
Rivera, G. *et al.* (1986). *New Engl. J. Med.* **315**, 273–278.
Schauer, P. *et al.* (1983). *J. Clin. Oncol.* **1**, 462–470.

CHRONIC LYMPHOCYTIC LEUKEMIA

Full details of the single agent therapy are not given here. See drug details.

SINGLE AGENTS

Chlorambucil
This can be used as *continuous therapy* as a daily dose, usually *2 mg/day* after initiation of treatment with *0·1–0·2 mg/kg* for 3–6 weeks or *as intermittent therapy*, employing 15–25 mg/day for 4–5 days every 3–4 weeks, with or without the addition of 40–60 mg prednisone PO for the same period.

Cyclophosphamide
2–4 mg/kg/day PO for 10 days followed by adjustment of the dose for continued therapy, according to the response.

Fludarabine monophosphate (see text on p. 42).
Cycles of 20–25 mg/m^2 IV during days 1–5. No treatment during days 6–28. For 6–12 cycles if responding.

Reference
M.J. Keating *et al.* (1988) *Leukemia* **2:** 157–164.

α-Interferon
This can be used at 3 x 10^6 i.u./m^2/day or 3 x per week. Usually after stable disease achieved.

Reference
C. Rozman, E. Montserrat *et al* (1988) *Blood*: **5,** 1295.
G.A. Pangalis & E. Griva (1988) *Cancer* **61**: 869.

COMBINATION CHEMOTHERAPY FOR CLL

CAP

Cyclophosphamide	750 mg/m^2	IV	day 1
Adriamycin*	50 mg/m^2	IV	day 1
Prednisone	100 mg/day	PO	days 1–5

No treatment given from day 6–21.
Courses repeated until CR achieved, followed by maintenance* for 18 months, using cyclophosphamide and prednisone only.

*Adriamycin given to a maximum cumulative dose of 450 mg/m^2 (9 courses).

Reference
Keating M.J. *et al.* (1990). *Leukemia and Lymphoma* **2**, 391–397.

CHOP

Cyclophosphamide	300 mg/m^2	IV	days 1–5
Vincristine	1 mg/m^2	IV	day 1
Doxorubicin	25 mg/m^2	IV	day 1
Prednisone	40 mg/m^2	PO	days 1–5

No treatment given from days 6–28. Treatment is given for 6 months followed by 6 more every 3 months. Total treatment for 2 years.

Reference
Binet *et al.* (1989). *Brit. J. Haem.* **43**, 334–340.

M-2 (BCMVP)

Given as for multiple myeloma. (p 127)

Reference
Kempin, S. *et al.* (1982). *Blood* **60**, 110–1121.

POACH

Prednisone	100 mg/day	PO	days 1–7
Vincristine	2 mg/m^2	IV	day 1
Ara-C	24 mg/m^2	IV	q. 12 h on days 1–5
Cyclophosphamide	500 mg/m^2	IV	day 1
Adriamycin*	15 mg/m^2	IV	days 1, 8 and 5

No treatment given on days 16–28. 3–9 cycles are given depending on response and whether CR is achieved. After CR two more courses are given and thereafter treatment is stopped.

*Adriamycin given to a maximum cumulative dose of 450 mg/m^2 (9 courses).

Reference

Keating, M.J. *et al.* (1988). *Leukemia* **2**, 157–164.

CHRONIC MYELOID LEUKEMIA AND BLAST TRANSFORMATION

Full details of the oral therapy for CML are not given and are provided under the drug details. Some of the regimens for treating transformed CML are given.

SINGLE AGENTS IN CML

Busulfan PO daily, see page 26
Hydroxyurea PO daily, see page 44
α-Interferon SC, see page 47

COMBINED REGIMENS

Blast transformation of CML

In general, if predominantly ***Lymphoid crisis:***

Prednisone 60 mg/m^2/day PO
Vincristine 0·03 mg/kg/day IV, weekly
Adriamycin and L-asparaginase may also be added as in ALL.
6-MP at 2·5 mg/kg/day may also be given, daily or thrice weekly PO as maintenance.

If predominantly ***Myeloid (ANLL) crisis:***

Daunomycin, Ara-C ± 6-TG may be given but other protocols have been tried. (see ANLL)

High-dose Ara-C with or without Busulfan

High-dose Ara-C 3 g/m^2 IV q.12 h for 3 days (days 1–3).
No treatment for one week on days 4–10.
If the marrow is still cellular this is followed by a second course of *high-dose Ara-C* 3 g/m^2 IV q.12 h for 3 days.

Patients who had cryopreserved marrow available received the above regimen followed by autologous bone-marrow infusion. If marrow was still cellular after the completion of the Ara-C, Busulfan 4 mg/kg/day was given for 4 days followed by marrow infusion two days later.

Reference

Preisler, H.D. *et al.* (1984). *Cancer Treat. Rep.* **68,** 1351–1355.

5-Azacytidine and VP-16

5-Azacytidine	150 mg/m^2	IV	days 1–5, given every 8 h in 3 divided doses
VP-16	75 mg/m^2		days 1–5

No treatment given on days 6–21.

Reference

Schiffer, C.A. *et al.* (1982). *Cancer Treat. Rep.* **66,** 267–271.

DATA

Daunomycin	10 mg/m^2	IV	days 1–5
5-Azacytidine	150 mg/m^2		days 1–5 given every 8 h in 3 divided doses
6-TG	75 mg/m^2	PO	q.12 h, days 1–5
Ara-C	75 mg/m^2	PO	q.12 h, days 1–5

Reference

Winton, E.F. *et al.* (1981). *Canc. Treat. Rep.* **65,** 389–392.

DAV(T)

Daunomycin	25 mg/m^2	IV	days 2 and 3
Ara-C	75 mg/m^2	IV	over 24 h, days 1–5
VP-16	100 mg/m^2	IV	over 2 days 4–5
or			
6-TG	100 mg/m^2	PO	days 1–5

Reference

Anger, B. and Heimpel, H. (1989). *Blut* **58,** 299–301.

DVPA

Doxorubicin	30 mg	IV	days 1–3
Vincristine	2 mg	IV	day 1
Prednisone	40 mg/m^2	PO	days 1–6
Ara-C	100 mg/m^2	IV	continuous days 5–7
or			
High-dose Ara-C	3 g/m^2	IV	q.12 h days 5–7

If cryopreserved autologous chronic phase bone-marrow was available it was infused on day 10.

Reference

Preisler, H.D. *et al.* (1984). *Cancer Treat. Rep.* **68,** 1351–1355.

Mithramycin and Hydroxyurea

Mithramycin 25 μg/kg IV every other day for 3 weeks
and
Hydroxurea 1·5–4·0 g/day PO depending on the WBC count (If WBC $> 100 \times 10^9$, 4 g/day; 75–100 $\times 10^9$, 3 g/day; 50–75 $\times 10^9$, 2 g/day; 15–50 $\times 10^9$, 1–1·5 g/day; 7·5–15 $\times 10^9$, 0·5 g/day).

If there is clinical response, the next cycle should use mithramycin 25 μg/kg 1–3 × per week and daily hydroxyurea, as above.

Reference

Koller, C.A. and Miller, D.M. (1986). *New Engl. J. Med.* **315,** 1433.

TRAMPCOL

6-TG	100 mg/m^2	PO	days 3–5
Rubidomycin (Daunorubicin)	25 mg/m^2	IV	day 1
Ara-C	100 mg/m^2	IV	days 3–5
MTX	7·5 mg/m^2	IV	days 3–5
Prednisone	200 mg	PO	days 1–5
Cyclophosphamide	100 mg/m^2	IV	days 3–5
Oncovin	2 mg	IV	day 1
L-Asparaginase	8000 i.u./m^2	IV	days 1–28

Reference

Spiers, A.S.D. *et al.* (1974). *Brit. Med. Journal* **3,** 77–80.

SOME PREPARATORY REGIMENS FOR CYTOREDUCTION IN AUTOLOGOUS BMT

Some selected regimens used for autologous ABMT in hematological neoplasia. For full details see references provided at the end of this selection. Obviously, many different centers are using their own regimens and we only include a few examples.

BAC

BCNU	300 mg/m^2	IV	day 1
Ara-C	200 mg/m^2	IV	days 2–5
Cyclophosphamide	35 mg/kg or 1·5 mg/m^2	IV	days 1–4 infused over 30 min.

BACAT

BCNU	300 mg/m^2	IV	day 1
Adriamycin	50 mg/m^2	IV	day 1
Cyclophosphamide	1500 mg/m^2	IV	days 1–3
Ara-C	100 mg/m^2	IV	b.d. on days 1–4
6-TG	100 mg/m^2	IV	b.d. on days 1–4

BACT

BCNU	200 mg/m^2	IV	day 1 10–60 min
Ara-C	200 mg/m^2	IV	continuous 30 min days 2–5
Cyclophosphamide	50 mg/kg	IV	30 min days 2–5
6-TG	200 mg/m^2	PO	q.12 h days 2–5

BAM

BCNU	300 mg/m^2	IV	day 1
Ara-C	200 mg/m^2	IV	days 1–4
MTX	1000 mg/m^2		day 1

BAVM

BCNU	300 mg/m^2	IV	over 60 min on day 1
Ara-C	200 mg/m^2	IV	over 12 h or as a 30 min infusion, on days 22–5
Vindesine	1·3 mg/m^2	IV	continuously over 24 h days 2–5
Melphalan	140 mg/m^2		infusion over 5 min on day 6

BEA

BCNU	300 mg/m^2	IV	infused over 30–60 min on day 1
Etoposide	250 mg/m^2	IV	infused over 60 min on days 1–4
Ara-C	200 mg/m^2	IV	over 30 min or 12 h infusion on days 2–5

BEAC

BCNU	300 mg/m^2	IV	day 1
Etoposide	75 mg/m^2	IV	days 1–4
Ara-C	200 mg/m^2	IV	days 1–4
Cyclophosphamide	1500 mg/m^2		days 1–4

BEAM

BCNU	300 mg/m^2	IV	infused over 60 min on day 1
Etoposide	100–200 mg/m^2	IV	days 2–5
Ara-C	200–400 mg/m^2		days 2–5
Melphalan	140 mg/m^2		day 6

BEC

BCNU	300 mg/m^2	IV	infused over 60 min on day 1.
Etoposide*	100 mg/m^2	IV	q.12 h on days 1–3.
Cyclophosphamide	1·5 g/m^2	IV	infused over 30 min on days 1–4.

*Can be escalated and given as 250 mg/m^2 infused over 60 min.

BECAM

BCNU	300 mg/m^2	IV	day 1
Etoposide	200 mg/m^2	IV	days 2–5
Cyclophosphamide	60 mg/kg	IV	day 4
Ara-C	200 mg/m^2	IV	days 3–6
Melphalan	60–90 mg/m^2		day 5–6

CMEC

Carmustine	800 mg/m^2		day 1
Mitoxantrone	12–18 mg/m^2	IV	days 2–4
Etoposide	150–300 mg/m^2	IV	days 2–4
Ara-C	300 mg/m^2	IV	days 2–4

HiBU ± C

Busulfan 16 mg/kg in 4 daily doses i.e. 1 mg/kg PO given every 6 h for 16 doses (days 1–4) with or without Cyclophosphamide 50 mg/kg IV for 4 days (days 5–8)
Autologous BMT on day 10.

HiME

High-dose melphalan alone IV 180–200 mg/m^2 infusion given over 5 min.

SELECTED REFERENCES

Armitage, J.O. *et al.* (1986). *Europ. J. Cancer Clin. Oncol.* **22,** 871.
Armitage, J.O. *et al.* (1986). *Cancer Treat. Rep.* **70;** 871.
Champlin, R. and Gale, R.P. (1987). *Sem. Hematol.* **24,** 55.
Champlin, R. and Gale, R.P. (1987). *Blood* **69,** 1551.
Gore M. *et al.* (1989). *Lancet,* 14 October, 879–882.
Gorin, N.C. *et al.* (1985). *Europ. J. Cancer Clin. Oncol.* **20,** 217.
Gorin, N.C. *4th EBMTG Survey Bone Marrow Transplantation Suppl.* **2,** 320.
McMillan, A.K. *et al.* (1990). *Leukemia and Lymphoma* **1,** 157.
Phillip, T. *et al.* (1983). *Europ. J. Cancer Clin. Oncol.* **119,** 1871.
Phillip, T. *et al.* (1984). *Lancet* **1,** 391.
Phillip T. *et al.* (1984). *New Engl. J. Med.* **310,** 1557.
Phillip T. *et al.* (1985). *Brit. J. Haematol.* **60,** 599.
Phillip, T. *et al.* (1986). *J. Clin. Oncol.* **4,** 4809.
Phillip, T., Armitage, J.O. *et al.* (1987). *New Engl. J. Med.* **316,** 1493.
Singer, J.R. and Goldstone, A.H. (1986). *Clin. Haematol.* **15,** 105.
Takavorian, T., Canellos, G.P. *et al.* (1987). *New Engl. J. Med.* **316,** 1499.
Verndonck L.F. *et al.* (1985). *Blood* **65,** 984.

PROTOCOL INDEX

MINE
MIV
VEMP
VP-I-P

Undifferentiated/Lymphoblastic or Burkitt's Lymphoma

NIH example
Stanford University Medical School example
APO

Multiple Myeloma

ABCP
Alkeran
High-dose Alkeran + ABMT
CAP-BAP
Recombinant α-Interferon
M2 Regimen
Methylprednisolone
VAD
VAMP
VBAP
VBMCP
VCAD-VAD
VCAP

Acute Leukemia

ANLL
ADOAP
COAP
DAT
DOAP
Epirubicin and Ara-C
GAC (using methyl GAG)
IAE
Idarubicin and Ara-C
m-AMSA and Ara-C
Mitoxantrone and Ara-C
OAP
POMP
ROAP
VAPA

Acute Promyelocytic Leukemia (M3, FAB)

Regimens for Relapsed or Refractory ANLL
DAC
HiDAC and *m*-AMSA/ mitoxantrone/idarubicin/ epirubicin/l-asparaginase
HiDA ASNASE
Idarubicin + Ara-C
VP-16 + IDAC
VP-16 and 5-Azacytidine

Example of a regimen used in MRC trial for AML

Induction and Consolidation Regimens
DA and DAC
MAZE

ALL
L-10 Type ALL protocol (older protocol)
ALL protocol (standard risk)
European style adult ALL protocol (high-risk)
Another recent regimen used for treating adult ALL
High/Intermediate-dose Ara-C

Chronic Lymphocytic Leukemia

CAP
Chlorambucil
CHOP
Cyclophosphamide
Deoxycoformycin
Fludarabine phosphate
α-Interferon
M-2 BCMVP
POACH

Chronic Myeloid Leukemia and Blast Transformation

High-dose Ara-C with or without Busulfan
5-Azacytidine – VP16
DATA
DAV(T)
DVPA
Hydroxyurea
α-Interferon
Mithramycin and Hydroxyurea
TRAMPCOL

Some Preparatory Regimens for Cytoreduction in ABMT

BAC
BACAT
BACT
BAM
BAVM
BEA
BEAC
BEAM
BEC
BECAM
CMEC
HIBU±C
HiME